Electronic Resources in Medical Libraries: Issues and Solutions

Electronic Resources in Medical Libraries: Issues and Solutions has been co-published simultaneously as *Journal of Electronic Resources in Medical Libraries*, Volume 4, Numbers 1/2 2007.

Electronic Resources in Medical Libraries: Issues and Solutions

Elizabeth Connor, MLS, AHIP
M. Sandra Wood, MLS, MBA, AHIP, FMLA
Editors

Electronic Resources in Medical Libraries: Issues and Solutions has been co-published simultaneously as *Journal of Electronic Resources in Medical Libraries*, Volume 4, Numbers 1/2 2007.

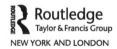

Routledge
Taylor & Francis Group
NEW YORK AND LONDON

First Published by

The Haworth Press, Inc., 10 Alice Street, Binghamton, NY 13904-1580

Transferred to Digital Printing 2009 by Routledge
711 Third Avenue, New York NY 10017
2 Park Square, Milton Park, Abingdon, Oxon, OX14 4RN

Routledge is an imprint of the Taylor & Francis Group, an informa business

First issued in paperback 2012

Electronic Resources in Medical Libraries: Issues and Solutions has been co-published simultaneously as *Journal of Electronic Resources in Medical Libraries*™, Volume 4, Numbers 1/2 2007.

The development, preparation, and publication of this work has been undertaken with great care. However, the publisher, employees, editors, and agents of The Haworth Press and all imprints of The Haworth Press, Inc., including The Haworth Medical Press® and Pharmaceutical Products Press®, are not responsible for any errors contained herein or for consequences that may ensue from use of materials or information contained in this work. With regard to case studies, identities and circumstances of individuals discussed herein have been changed to protect confidentiality. Any resemblance to actual persons, living or dead, is entirely coincidental.

The Haworth Press is committed to the dissemination of ideas and information according to the highest standards of intellectual freedom and the free exchange of ideas. Statements made and opinions expressed in this publication do not necessarily reflect the views of the Publisher, Directors, management, or staff of The Haworth Press, Inc., or an endorsement by them.

Library of Congress Cataloging-in-Publication Data

Electronic resources in medical libraries : issues and solutions / Elizabeth Connor, M. Sandra Wood, editors.
    p. cm.
    "Co-published simultaneously as Journal of electronic resources in medical libraries, volume 4, numbers 1/2."
    Includes bibliographical references and index.
    ISBN-13: 978-0-7890-3513-4 (hbk)
    ISBN-13: 978-0-4155-4272-2 (pbk)
    1. Medical libraries–Collection development. 2. Medicine–Electronic information resources. 3. Libraries–Special collections–Electronic information resources 4. Libraries–Special collections–Electronic journals. 5. Libraries and electronic publishing. I. Connor, Elizabeth, MLS. II. Wood, M. Sandra. III. Journal of electronic resources in medical libraries.
    Z675.M4E44 2007
    025.2'84–dc22

                                       2006039152

Electronic Resources in Medical Libraries: Issues and Solutions

CONTENTS

ABOUT THE EDITORS

Elizabeth Connor, MLS, AHIP, is Assistant Professor of Library Science and Science Liaison at the Daniel Library of the Citadel, the Military College of South Carolina in Charleston. A distinguished member of the Academy of Health Information Professionals, she has held library leadership positions at major teaching hospitals and academic medical centers in Maryland, Saudi Arabia, Connecticut, South Carolina, and the Commonwealth of Dominica.

Ms. Connor has authored several peer-reviewed articles about electronic resources, women's health information, science search engines, chat reference, and medical informatics, and has published more than 70 book reviews in *Library Journal, Against the Grain, Bulletin of the Medical Library Association, Journal of the Medical Library Association, Medical Reference Services Quarterly, Doody's Reviews*, and *The Post & Courier.*

Ms. Connor manages the book review process for *Medical Reference Services Quarterly* and is co-editor of *Journal of Electronic Resources in Medical Libraries.*

Ms. Connor is the author of *Internet Guide to Travel Health* and *Internet Guide to Food Safety and Security;* and editor of *A Guide to Developing End User Education Programs in Medical Libraries* and *Planning, Renovating, and Constructing Library Facilities in Hospitals, Academic Medical Centers, and Health Organizations,* all published by The Haworth Press, Inc. She is the editor of a forthcoming series of textbooks for library school students, also to be published by The Haworth Press, Inc.

M. Sandra Wood, MLS, MBA, AHIP, FMLA, is Librarian Emerita, Pennsylvania State University. Previously, she was Librarian, Reference and Database Services, The George T. Harrell Library, The Milton S. Hershey Medical Center, The Pennsylvania State University College of Medicine, Hershey, PA. She has over 35 years of experience as a medical reference librarian, with experience/interests in general reference, management of reference services, database and Internet searching, and user instruction. Ms. Wood has been widely published in the field of medical reference and is Editor of *Medical Reference Services Quarterly, Journal of Consumer Health on the Internet*, and Co-editor of the *Journal of Electronic Resources in Medical Libraries* (Haworth). She is author of the Haworth book, *Internet Guide to Cosmetic Surgery for Women*, published in 2005, and *Internet Guide to Cosmetic Surgery for Men*, published in 2006, and is editor or co-editor of several other Haworth books, including *Women's Health on the Internet, Health Care Resources on the Internet: A Guide for Librarians and Health Care Consumers, Men's Health on the Internet*, and *Cancer Resources on the Internet*. She is a member of the Medical Library Association and the Special Libraries Association, and has served on the MLA's Board of Directors as Treasurer. Ms. Wood is also a Fellow of the Medical Library Association.

Introduction

Elizabeth Connor

M. Sandra Wood

As health care professionals, researchers, educators, and students rely increasingly on digital content to learn new information, collaborate, and disseminate research results, effective acquisition and management of e-resources have become essential functions for all organizational units of a medical library including administration, collection development, cataloging, reference, instruction, interlibrary loan, outreach, and information technology. The complexities of choosing and authenticating electronic journals and books for campus and off-campus users have replaced the challenges involved with ordering, processing, and cataloging print journals and books. Although some of these issues are specific to medical libraries, most are relevant to all types of libraries, from academic and special libraries, to public and school libraries. All libraries provide access to electronic resources and while their solutions to some issues may depend on local situations, issues such as licensing, usage statistics, and pricing are universal.

Electronic Resources in Medical Libraries: Issues and Solutions brings together a unique collection of papers dealing with issues surrounding electronic access and utilization of books and journals, including collection development, pricing, open access, licensing, remote access, statistics, publisher liability, and the Semantic Web. Many of the articles actually present solutions for some of these issues; others describe the issues

---

[Haworth co-indexing entry note]: "Introduction." Connor, Elizabeth, and M. Sandra Wood. Co-published simultaneously in the *Journal of Electronic Resources in Medical Libraries* (The Haworth Information Press, an imprint of The Haworth Press, Inc.) Vol. 4, No. 1/2, 2007, pp. 1-3; and: *Electronic Resources in Medical Libraries: Issues and Solutions* (ed: Elizabeth Connor, and M. Sandra Wood) The Haworth Information Press, an imprint of The Haworth Press, Inc., 2007, pp. 1-3. Single or multiple copies of this article are available for a fee from The Haworth Document Delivery Service [1-800-HAWORTH, 9:00 a.m. - 5:00 p.m. (EST). E-mail address: docdelivery@haworthpress.com].

without simple solutions. Examples are drawn from medical libraries, both academic and hospital, and include not only U.S. libraries, but libraries in Qatar, Latin America, and the Caribbean. Access to electronic resources is, indeed, a worldwide issue.

These ten articles represent a variety of approaches, situations, and challenges. In "Moving the Big Deal," Chung Sook Kim and Barbara M. Koehler discuss how the William H. Welch Library at Johns Hopkins has entered into several Big Deals, helping to alleviate financial problems while expanding access to the biomedical literature. They detail licensing issues along with consortium purchasing, and how the Big Deal has helped keep costs level while increasing the number of journals. Maggie Wineburgh-Freed overviews pricing models and the evolution of electronic journal pricing, and also discusses implications of open access publishing in her article, "Scholarly E-Journal Pricing Models and Open Access Publishing." Open access may be one way to help keep journal costs low for libraries. In their discussion of electronic resource licensing, "Extending Electronic Resource Licenses to a Newly Established Overseas Medical School Branch," Michael A. Wood, Carole Thompson, and Kristine M. Alpi describe the efforts and benefits to users to extend contracts and licenses to electronic resources that are available at the Weill Cornell Medical College in New York City and the main University Library of Cornell University in Ithaca, New York, to the newly established Weill Cornell Medical College in Qatar. Access, cost, and licensing are among the major issues that needed to be resolved to provide equal access to electronic resources to medical students in Doha, Qatar. Access to electronic health information is the major issue described by C. Verônica Abdala and Rosane Taruhn in their paper, "Access to Health Information in Latin America and the Caribbean." The authors describe the Virtual Health Library (VHL), HINARI, and other cooperative efforts in Latin America and the Caribbean.

Rick Ralston analyzed online journal use at Indiana University School of Medicine via statistics provided by the journal vendor and through Web site linking. In "Assessing Online Use: Are Statistics from Web-Based Online Journal Lists Representative?," he concludes that the usage counts were not accurate enough to be used for journal cancellation decisions. In "Two Interfaces, One Knowledge Base: The Development of a Combined E-Journal Web Page," Felicia Yeh and Karen McMullen describe the efforts of the libraries of the University of South Carolina system to combine their e-journal list with that of the School of Medicine Library. Their solution involved an electronic resource management system, TDNet. Julie A. Garrison and Pamela A. Grudzien investigated how electronic journal usage affected the full-service document delivery available of off-campus students at Central Michigan University, in "Off-Campus User Behavior: Are They Finding Electronic Journals on Their Own or Still Ordering Through Document Delivery?" Document delivery requests have decreased while online usage has increased. In "Integrating E-Resources into an Online Catalog: The Hospital Library Experience," Devica Samsundar describes how the Baptist Health South Florida libraries migrated to a Web-based online catalog for access to their e-resources. The successful project is detailed from the planning stage through its completion.

A. Bruce Strauch, Earl Walker, and Mark Bebensee discuss publisher and products liability in their paper, "Is There a Pending Change in Medical Publisher and Library Liability?" As the distinction between publisher and producer/creator blurs with online resources, both libraries and vendors will need to be more aware of liability issues. Jon C. Ferguson describes the Semantic Web and applications to digital libraries in "Semantic Web Technologies: Opportunities for Domain Targeted Libraries?" His examples were derived from The Initiative for Maternal Mortality Programme Assessment (IMMPACT).

These and other issues will continue to vex and challenge all librarians, not just medical librarians, as present-day hybrid collections evolve into totally electronic environments. Electronic resources–whether books, journals, databases, Web sites, or combinations of these–present new and different issues to both librarians and producers/publishers. These papers offer some solutions to the issues surrounding electronic resources, and indicate areas for further research.

Moving the Big Deal

Chung Sook Kim
Barbara M. Koehler

SUMMARY. Shifting collections from print to electronic materials has been costly and challenging. The Big Deal collection of journals offered one way to consolidate costs and provide wide access. The William H. Welch Library at Johns Hopkins University entered into several Big Deals to provide users with electronic materials but faced serious problems in financing such items. By entering into collaborative arrangements with other Johns Hopkins libraries and eventually with a consortium, the Welch Library was able to maintain its same level of serials expenditures while dramatically increasing access to a wide spectrum of journals. doi:10.1300/ J383v04n01_02 *[Article copies available for a fee from The Haworth Document Delivery Service: 1-800-HAWORTH. E-mail address: <docdelivery@haworthpress.com> Website: <http://www.HaworthPress.com> © 2007 by The Haworth Press, Inc. All rights reserved.]*

KEYWORDS. Electronic resources, electronic journals, Big Deal, library collections, collection development, consortia, licensing, funding

---

Chung Sook Kim (csk@jhmi.edu) is Associate Director for Digital Library Services, and Barbara M. Koehler (bmk@jhmi.edu) is Publications Specialist; both at Welch Medical Library, Johns Hopkins University, 1900 East Monument Street, Baltimore, MD 21205.

[Haworth co-indexing entry note]: "Moving the Big Deal." Kim, Chung Sook, and Barbara M. Koehler. Co-published simultaneously in the *Journal of Electronic Resources in Medical Libraries* (The Haworth Information Press, an imprint of The Haworth Press, Inc.) Vol. 4, No. 1/2, 2007, pp. 5-14; and: *Electronic Resources in Medical Libraries: Issues and Solutions* (ed: Elizabeth Connor, and M. Sandra Wood) The Haworth Information Press, an imprint of The Haworth Press, Inc., 2007, pp. 5-14. Single or multiple copies of this article are available for a fee from The Haworth Document Delivery Service [1-800-HAWORTH, 9:00 a.m. - 5:00 p.m. (EST). E-mail address: docdelivery@haworthpress.com].

Available online at http://jerml.haworthpress.com
© 2007 by The Haworth Press, Inc. All rights reserved.
doi:10.1300/J383v04n01_02

INTRODUCTION

Over the years, collection development has evolved from the acquisition and maintenance of paper to the development of the fully electronic collection. In the early stages of this metamorphosis, libraries and publishers sought ways to ease the pain of monumental change. Licensing individual electronic titles individually quickly overwhelmed libraries and publishers. Once the electronic journal became a popular reality, publishers grappled with their own changes, and sought new ways to market, distribute, and charge for their collections. Out of those deliberations came the Big Deal, which simplified the subscription process for both the library and the publisher. The Big Deal is an aggregation of journals that publishers sell as a unit with one price. Libraries license electronic access to all of a publisher's journals at a cost based on their current payments plus an additional fee. Price increases are capped for a number of years. The Big Deal usually allows the library to cancel paper subscriptions at some savings or offer additional paper subscriptions at discounted prices. However, content is bundled so that individual journal subscriptions can no longer be cancelled in their electronic format.[1] The Big Deal is commended for encouraging library users' quick acceptance of electronic content.[2] But these packages have often been a source of frustration to libraries, forcing them to pay for titles they may not want, even though they do offer users access to a wide range of titles for one inclusive fee. Whether librarians like it or not, the Big Deal has been a necessary part of the electronic landscape. At the William H. Welch Library at Johns Hopkins University, several large packages of electronic journals, Big Deals, have constituted the bulk of the online journal collection.

HISTORY

The Welch Medical Library, founded in 1929 to serve the schools of medicine and public health and the Johns Hopkins Hospital, is situated on the East Baltimore campus of The Johns Hopkins University. Over the years, service was expanded to include the School of Nursing and several other affiliated groups that constitute the Johns Hopkins Health System. Users of the Johns Hopkins Medical Institutions enjoy abundant electronic resources (over 36,000 titles from all university libraries) anywhere, anytime. When they search PubMed or any other bibliographic database, they can click full-text buttons for instant access to articles. If there are no full-text links, articles can be requested and delivered to their desktops within a short period of time. A comment from a Hopkins professor of Cardiology expresses the general sentiment of Welch users: "... the on-line service Welch provides–one of the crown jewels of JHMI ... you do have a great collection whose availability, 24/day, is a shining example of Hopkins' greatness...."

Welch staff members have been planning their electronic future for over 25 years. The seed was planted by Richard A. Polacsek, who served as the library's fourth director from 1969 to 1984. In 1980, he bought a minicomputer and initiated the development that led to Welch's Integrated Library System online catalog in 1983. The computerization of operations was a *conditio sine qua non* for the future of the Welch Medical Library, the information resource center for the entire medical campus.

Nina Matheson, library director from 1984 to 1993, built on Dr. Polacsek's beginnings, adding databases including MiniMedline in 1985, TOXNET in 1988, and by 1993, MEDLINE 500 +, WelCORK (the Dartmouth CORK alcohol database), and Hopkins Current Contents®. This laid the foundation on which a large electronic collection would be built. In 1996, Welch began that collection with the purchase of 15 e-journals from Ovid and eight databases. By 1999, the collection had grown to include 12 databases and 236 e-journals.

FUNDING

Welch moved forward with the benefit of cutting edge technology, but another necessary component to growth was funding support from the schools that used the collections. The Welch Library has been funded over the years by the School of Medicine, School of Public Health, School of Nursing, and Johns Hopkins Hospital. For the last 20 years, these groups were assessed according to their use of Welch services. As the library's collection migrated from print materials to electronic, there was a growing need to increase funding in order to purchase costly databases as well as large and very expensive packages of journals. Thoughtful decisions were made to allocate funds wisely for acquisition of as many e-resources as possible, but often the funding did not keep up with increases in journal prices nor allow for the purchase of the many new resources offered online. Welch struggled to find money to expand its electronic collection. Along the way, the decision was made to drop Ovid MEDLINE and move to the National Library of

Medicine's free Grateful Med, using the money saved to purchase more titles. This move, initially controversial with users, allowed the library to purchase hundreds more e-journals. The welcome increase in the collection more than compensated for the loss of the popular Ovid search engine.

LICENSING THE BIG DEALS

In 2000, Nancy Roderer was appointed director of Welch Library. Her in-depth analysis revealed that the collection had suffered from the cuts and too modest budget increases of the 1990s. Ms. Roderer urged library funding sources to provide more collection money in the coming years. They agreed, and Welch staff created a Five Year Collection Plan (FY2001/02-FY2005/06), subsequently approved by the library committee, that provided substantial funding until 2006. The first five-year plan in FY02 resulted in users gaining access to more than 3,700 print and e-journals. Approximately 90% of all Welch's journals were online with 370 journals left in print. In each year of the plan, about 10% more money was requested to cover renewals and to add new titles. Thanks to the increased collection budget, e-resources grew from 248 titles to 1,800 titles (+628%) within one year.

Subsequently, a second Five Year Collection Plan (FY07-FY11) was drafted and approved by the library's funding sources. The second five-year plan included an overall annual inflation rate of 11% with adjustments downward for increases in open access journals and upward for backfiles.

The two plans were developed based on the following goals:

- Order all materials in electronic format if available; order print materials when print is the only choice.
- Meet the demand for broader subject access with e-resources.
- Meet the demand for cross-campus access with e-resources.
- Continue to expand the number of e-books as they become available.
- Continue to expand the number of databases. (This is the most rapidly growing area of resources, as publishers experiment with new methods of packaging).
- License online reference books and online reference databases.
- Maintain one print journal copy among the JHU libraries until archival issues are resolved.

- Add necessary print books each year until more are available electronically.
- Work with publishers to develop usage statistics for electronic materials.
- Cancel print journals that are available electronically: 10% of current subscription titles in Y02, 20% in Y03, 20% in Y04, 20% in Y05, and 20% in Y06.
- Supplement the collection with free interlibrary loan for other subject areas.
- Weed print book collection of editions that were published before 1985.
- Weed journal collection of any ceased or dead journal titles published before 1985.
- Offer weeded materials to the Institute of the History of Medicine or transfer to the remote storage facility.

From the very beginning, Welch's goal was to provide access to e-resources remotely since twenty-first century users expect 24/7 access. Beginning in 2001, the library started to license e-journals only and stopped subscribing to print duplicates. Print was purchased when there was no electronic option. Welch experimented with the new paradigm, the Big Deal, licensing packages such as Kluwer Academic journals through the PALINET Library Network and IDEAL through the CIRLA (Chesapeake Information and Research Library Alliance) consortium. The advantage to joining the fledgling PALINET consortium was that the library paid PALINET only for its subscribed titles, but it could access the publisher's whole list of titles. The library also licensed collections from, Ovid, Cell Press, SciFinder, FirstSearch, STAT!Ref, ScienceDirect®, Web of Science, and MDConsult.

As the library acquired more electronic titles, it became apparent that users from all Hopkins units were eager to look at e-journals from all Hopkins libraries. Licensing an e-journal for just one location was no longer practical. Staff quickly realized that Welch had to license titles for all Hopkins locations as one site, a concept that was irrelevant in the era of print. As librarians from various sites met and discussed the issues, they realized that it would be beneficial to license certain packages together and to share the costs. How to pay for these huge electronic products was on everyone's mind. Cost sharing provided a way to extend budgeted funds, seeking the best deals possible with the pooled money.

The Milton S. Eisenhower Library on the main Hopkins campus initially shared costs with Welch for FirstSearch, SciFinder, and Web of Science®. In 2002, Welch purchased 142 titles from Harcourt Health Sciences, Lippincott, Mary Ann Liebert, UpToDate®, Wiley Current Protocols, and initiated a site license for Wiley Interscience®. The costs for Wiley Interscience were shared with the Eisenhower Library, and the licenses for all of the aforementioned items explicitly permitted use by all of Hopkins.

In 2003, Welch added Access Medicine, Ovid EMBASE 1980-, Wilson Web, and Dekker titles, sharing the cost with the Eisenhower Library with a formula for cost sharing that allowed the library with the main subject fields to pay the most. By this time, other Hopkins libraries had become aware of the advantages of providing materials for all of Hopkins and sharing the costs. In 2004, five Hopkins libraries agreed upon a formula based on each library's collection budget. That year, 27 more e-resources were added with the libraries sharing the costs, among them: JSTOR, *Nature* titles, Science, IEEE journals, LexisNexis®, Maryland Digital Library, and EBSCOhost®.

CONSORTIUM PURCHASING

Though cost sharing lessened the financial burden on each library, bigger savings was possible through consortial purchasing of the Big Deals. At the same time, consortial purchases would dramatically increase the number of titles to which any one library alone could provide access. Typically, the consortium required the library to pay only for its own subscribed titles. However, the consortial arrangement allowed the library access to the publisher's whole list. This was a win for both sides: the library had access to a greater number of titles for a relatively modest sum of money, and the publisher realized savings by dealing with one entity as opposed to several different libraries. Publishers secured guaranteed subscription fees from each library, issued one bill, and prepared one license agreement.

Hopkins libraries were interested in the NorthEast Research Libraries Consortium (NERL). NERL is a group of 27 academic research libraries and 45 affiliates whose common objectives are access and cost containment, joint licensing, and the possible joint deployment of electronic resources. Members share information about management and budgeting. NERL focuses on expensive (over $10K), scholarly e-resources that are important to research institutions. Their work is done mostly by volunteer members.[3] Within NERL, there are over 40 organizations that have some kind of health related activity, making this consortium an attractive option for Welch.

The Eisenhower Library joined NERL in 2003 and urged Welch to become part of the group. Because Welch had recently signed a two-year contract with Wiley, they were not eligible to join right away. Once that contract ended, Hopkins joined the NERL consortium in 2004 and was able to reduce their Wiley price cap by a comfortable margin. In addition, Hopkins users increased their access from 194 to about 350 journals, all Wiley titles published as of 2004.

Before renewing Wiley, ScienceDirect, and Springer titles in 2005, a study was done to see if the current subscription arrangement was cost-effective. Wiley was already in the second year of a contract with NERL. ScienceDirect titles were not part of NERL but were renewed annually with Elsevier due to the Eisenhower Library's desire to cancel some titles. Since Hopkins could not move ScienceDirect to NERL because of the cancellation history, they negotiated a three-year contract with Elsevier, saving a significant amount of money over a one-year contract. At the end of the current contract, Hopkins plans to add ScienceDirect to their NERL contract, which will substantially reduce their costs. That contract will allow Hopkins access to all ScienceDirect titles to which NERL subscribes. Access to the complete list of ScienceDirect titles requires that Hopkins subscribe to the Freedom Collection for an additional fee.

When the Springer package was available through NERL, Hopkins libraries left the PALINET consortium and added Springer titles to NERL since they would get a more favorable price cap for three years. The libraries had been paying a fee to a subscription agent and would lose some money, but the savings overall made the change worthwhile. Also, the libraries were given a one-time option to cancel up to 2% of the total cost before or during the contract years with NERL. Hopkins canceled all duplicate subscriptions. For print subscriptions, Hopkins pays the NERL fee plus received credits and postage/handling costs. Hopkins originally subscribed to about 490 titles but through NERL can access all 1,200 Springer titles.

In the future, the Hopkins libraries plan to license all e-resources as Hopkins site licenses, including the university's foreign locations. With the help of a consultant, the library cost sharing model will be revised to make it simpler and more equitable to each participating library.

OTHER LIBRARIES

What have other libraries done with regard to cost containment, collaboration, and consortial arrangements? Many libraries have chosen to opt out of some of their Big Deals because the aggregated cost was too high. Cornell, Harvard, University of Maryland, Duke, North Carolina State University, and the University of North Carolina–to name a few–opted out of the ScienceDirect Big Deal. The University of California (UC) renewed its subscription after some hard bargaining. The UC system wound up spending considerably less on their Elsevier journals as a result of their negotiations.[4]

The University of California system provides a useful model for other libraries interested in cost savings. The establishment of the California Digital Library (CDL) in the late 1990s led to a set of principles, one of which was to influence the marketplace through consortial purchasing. The CDL facilitated the purchase of large numbers of e-journals and databases with multi-year agreements that lowered the base cost for some large contracts. In several cases, the CDL was able to eliminate hyperinflation in the annual price increases sought by publishers. CDL principles and ground-breaking contracts echoed throughout libraries in North America. The University of California willingly and openly shared information about their tactics and negotiations with other libraries, inspiring others to try to influence the marketplace as well.[5]

Another large and diverse state consortium, OhioLINK, handled the Big Deal in a unique way. Because the Big Deal locks libraries into a package of journals with a contracted financial commitment over several years, it can cause problems when libraries have to manage static or shrinking budgets. OhioLINK has written into its consortial licenses a mechanism for gradual attrition of content and annual cost. Despite the Ohio consortium being so large and so varied, this mechanism appears to be a workable solution to the cost containment problem.[6]

Like Hopkins, Yale Library is already licensing all titles available through NERL and sharing the cost among libraries. Vanderbilt Library annually conducts a benchmarking study to collect information from other libraries in order to better manage their collection funds.

CONCLUSION

At one time not too long ago, each individual Hopkins library managed its own subscription list and persuaded its own funding groups to provide the necessary cash to support its collection. As computers increasingly intermingled university campuses and activities, the university's libraries realized that their fates were inextricably linked as were their budgets. To provide a resource for all of Hopkins meant a fresh look at collaboration for selection and funding arrangements. Initially, this led the libraries to the Big Deal. As costs continued to mount, the libraries agreed to adopt the cost sharing model that is currently in place. But they still sought a better model, one that would further reduce costs and still provide access to as many titles as possible. Moving the Big Deals to NERL is the answer for now, allowing the libraries to use their own home-grown cost-sharing model, to provide access to thousands of titles, and to maximize savings. Consortium licensing offers several benefits to the libraries:

- One license negotiation that covers any/all participants.
- Financial benefits include discounted prices; pooled financial resources for greater economy; capped price increases and budgetary stability; savings on interlibrary loan/document delivery and processing costs.
- One contact point for ordering and troubleshooting problems.
- Access to more titles.
- Timesaving for patrons who no longer have to wait for interlibrary loans and document delivery.

Welch Library staff are happy to share in these benefits and to realize savings that could not be realized by one library alone. Library consortia provide individual libraries with the opportunity for a new and rich collaboration. Though libraries have cooperated in a number of ways over time, consortial arrangements allow sharing in many new areas: building collections, managing resources, sharing costs, sharing expertise in computing, and digital preservation. This collaborative association may lead to other kinds of innovation beyond the pooling of money. Moving the Big Deals to a consortium has allowed the library to get more for its money. Together, libraries and publishers have worked out new pricing models that provide broader access to users, a step in the continuing evolution of scholarly publishing and user demands.

REFERENCES

1. Frazier, K. "The Librarian's Dilemma: Contemplating the Costs of the 'Big Deal.'" *D-Lib Magazine* 7(March 2001): Available: <http://www.dlib.org/dlib/march01/frazier/03frazier.html>. Accessed: June 14, 2006.

2. Rowse, M. "Consortial Purchasing: Time Runs Out for Unnatural Selection." Available: <http://www.researchinformation.info/riaut02consortialpurchasing.htm>. Accessed: June 13, 2006.

3. NERL Consortium Home Page. Available: <http://www.library.yale.edu/NERLpublic/>. Accessed: June 7, 2006.

4. ACRL Scholarly Communication Toolkit. Bundled or Aggregated Subscriptions to Electronic Journals. Available: <http://www.ala.org/ala/acrl/acrlissues/scholarlycomm/scholarlycommunicationtoolkit/faculty/facultyaggregation.htm>. Accessed: June 14, 2006.

5. SPARC Innovator University of California. Available: <http://www.arl.org/sparc/innovator/uc.html>. Accessed: July 26, 2006.

6. Gatten, J.N., and Sanville, T. "An Orderly Retreat from the Big Deal: Is It Possible for Consortia? " *D-Lib Magazine* 10(October 2004). Available: <http://www.dlib.org/dlib/october04/gatten/10gatten.html>. Accessed: August 18, 2006.

doi:10.1300/J383v04n01_02

Scholarly E-Journal Pricing Models and Open Access Publishing

Maggie Wineburgh-Freed

SUMMARY. This article provides an overview and description of the models being used to price electronic journals, reviews the development of electronic journals, and briefly discusses the history of journal pricing. The development and current situation of open-access scholarly publishing are also discussed. Open access may provide needed relief to the inexorable rise in journal prices, while increasing the impact of research distributed in this way. doi:10.1300/J383v04n01_03 *[Article copies available for a fee from The Haworth Document Delivery Service: 1-800- HAWORTH. E-mail address: <docdelivery@haworthpress.com> Website: <http://www. HaworthPress.com> © 2007 by The Haworth Press, Inc. All rights reserved.]*

KEYWORDS. Journal pricing, electronic journals, open access, open-access publishing, pricing models

---

Maggie Wineburgh-Freed, MLS, AHIP (mwfreed@usc.edu) is Associate Director for Collection Resources, Norris Medical Library, University of Southern California, 2003 Zonal Avenue, Los Angeles, CA 90089-9130.

[Haworth co-indexing entry note]: "Scholarly E-Journal Pricing Models and Open Access Publishing." Wineburgh-Freed, Maggie. Co-published simultaneously in the *Journal of Electronic Resources in Medical Libraries* (The Haworth Information Press, an imprint of The Haworth Press, Inc.) Vol. 4, No. 1/2, 2007, pp. 15-24; and: *Electronic Resources in Medical Libraries: Issues and Solutions* (ed: Elizabeth Connor, and M. Sandra Wood) The Haworth Information Press, an imprint of The Haworth Press, Inc., 2007, pp. 15-24. Single or multiple copies of this article are available for a fee from The Haworth Document Delivery Service [1-800-HAWORTH, 9:00 a.m. - 5:00 p.m. (EST). E-mail address: docdelivery@haworthpress.com].

INTRODUCTION

Publishers seek appropriate pricing models for electronic journals, but journal subscription prices in science, technology, and medical publishing continue to increase.[1, 2] The need to purchase electronic journals has taken more and more of health science libraries' collections budgets. A solution to this dilemma may be the increased availability of clinical and research literature in open-access articles and journals.

Birth and Development of Scholarly Electronic Journals

The first peer-reviewed full-text electronic journals began appearing in the 1980s and early 1990s, arising with the development of the Internet and the World Wide Web. Many of the earliest offerings were freely available on the Internet. The history and development of scholarly electronic journals have been well-documented in the literature,[3, 4] including a timeline of developments in the early days of electronic publishing.[5]

One of the earliest born-electronic journals in the health sciences was *Online Journal of Current Clinical Trials*, which began publication in 1992 as a joint venture of OCLC and the American Association for the Advancement of Science (AAAS). This journal used a unique graphical interface, GUIDON, which was developed by OCLC.[6] With the development of the World Wide Web in 1989 and its increased functionality, the technology became available to support more sophisticated publication and searching.[7]

Web-based electronic publishing and distribution began to grow at a rapid pace. A few early examples of electronic versions of well-respected biomedical titles include *Journal of Biological Chemistry*, which began to be co-published and hosted by Stanford University's HighWire Press in May 1995, and *Journal of Clinical Investigation*, published since 1926 by the American Society for Clinical Investigation, and made available online at no charge in January 1996. As electronic journals and the underlying technology have developed further, many features make them desirable to the academic and research community: faster processing and publishing, easy searchability, and the ability to link to supplementary material, including multimedia and remote access.

Since their beginnings ten to fifteen years ago, the number of scholarly titles made available via the Web has grown exponentially. Tenopir estimated in early 2004 that there were over 14,000 titles available online.[8] In a 2005 survey sponsored by the Association for Learned and

Professional Society Publishers (ALPSP), Cox found that 90% of journals are available in electronic versions.[9] Many publishers provide online access to their entire journal list, increasingly including digitized archives of their earliest issues.

EVOLUTION OF ELECTRONIC JOURNAL PRICING

Differentiated journal prices for individuals and institutions have existed for only the last 40 years. According to a 1977 study of print journals, in 1966 only 4% of periodicals had a dual pricing structure, and this had increased to just 15% by 1975.[10] How simple those times seem now, when the 1998 North American Serials Interest Group (NASIG) conference workshop discussed 16 different pricing models,[11] and Siar et al. cited an article that documents over 50 models.[12]

As electronic journal publishing began, publishers and distributors found many different methods of sustaining this new activity. In 1996, as part of the Open Journal Framework project, Hitchcock, Carr, and Hall produced a report that included information on the funding of early electronic journals, including those published commercially and non-commercially, and those that charged for subscriptions and those that did not.[13] The variety of funding sources and pricing models being used or proposed at that time were described, many of which are still being used today. They divided the publications into those that were electronic editions of existing journals and those that were electronic only titles and felt that the economics of the two types differed significantly. There were both commercial and non-commercial electronic only journals included in their study, although most of the commercial journals were supported by subscriptions. The authors were particularly concerned about the viability of electronic-only publications, because "... some electronic-only journals [are] supported by research or educational grants, and some by appropriate associations or societies, but by its nature this type of funding is often short-term, and the gap still has to be filled."[13] Even today that gap has not been adequately filled. A report recently produced by the Kaufman-Wills Group for the ALPSP found that:

> Over 40% of the Open Access journals are not yet covering their costs and, unlike subscription journals, there is no reason why the passage of time–evidenced in increasing submissions, quality or impact–should actually change that; their financial future therefore seems somewhat uncertain.[14]

As electronic journals have become more well-established, publishers explored a wide variety of pricing models to discover those that would be economically feasible. According to John Cox:

> The creation, testing, and evaluation of new business models is important in order to exploit the full potential of network technology. Publishers want to see their content reach all potential readers. The implication is that there may be a variety of pricing and access models to meet the usage needs and affordability criteria of different user communities.[15]

Some of the pricing models that have been used include: electronic-only journal free to all or for a set subscription price; electronic version of a print journal included with a print subscription for no additional fee; electronic version of a print journal included with a print subscription for a modest increment above the print subscription price; and separate and equal costs for print and/or electronic versions. In addition, several tiered pricing models not based on the print publication include: price per simultaneous user; price based on number of institutional FTEs; and price based on Carnegie classification (for academic institutions). Finally, packages or bundled subscriptions have been offered to individual institutions and to consortia or purchasing groups. These bundled subscriptions have frequently been based on the library's existing print and/or online only subscription list, usually with strict restrictions on cancellations.

All of these pricing models are currently in use, and frequently publishers have used more than one model successively. Each one has advantages and disadvantages, which are outlined in two reports from NASIG conferences in 1998[11] and 2005.[12] For example, the model based on the print subscription is fairly straightforward to manage, but may require retention of the print subscription when the library would prefer to subscribe to the electronic version only. Prices for a small number of simultaneous users may be lower than for unlimited access, but may cause difficulties with library patrons who are locked out from time to time. Prices based on Carnegie classification may seem unfair when the journal in question is a niche title, of interest to only a small number of faculty or researchers at an institution. Bundled titles may offer an advantageous price, but they do not allow librarians to choose titles that are of actual interest to the institution and may include subscriptions to poor quality titles.

OPEN-ACCESS PUBLISHING

Open-access publishing existed before the emergence of electronic journals as a method to distribute research findings promptly and widely, and partly in response to high journal prices. The author of this article defines open access generally, referring to "resources that are openly available to users with no requirements for authentication or payment."[16] In addition, it was often a way to take advantage of the emerging Internet and World Wide Web technology in a less restrictive format. One of the early entrants into the electronic publishing world was the Los Alamos National Laboratory's e-print arXiv which has provided a place for authors to self-archive their physics and mathematics articles since 1991.[17] This informal mode of scholarly communication serves researchers and scientists in their interactions with colleagues, one of the most important information-seeking behaviors. The open-access publishing model may include such informal self-archived sites; peer-reviewed journals with full open access, where all content is made immediately available at no charge; partial open access, where some content is held back or where some content is open and other content is by subscription; or delayed open access, where content is made freely available after an "embargo" period which may be months or years. For a more complete listing of types of open-access publishing, see table A-1 in Willinsky's book, *The Access Principle*.[18]

Authors and publishers alike have poorly understood open-access scholarly journals. First, there is the perception that all open-access scholarly journals are supported by author fees. As the Kaufman-Wills report for the ALPSP said:

> On the financial side, we were very surprised to find just how few of the Open Access journals raise any author-side charges at all; in fact, author charges are considerably more common (in the form of page charges, colour charges, reprint charges, etc.) among subscription journals.[14]

Open-access publishers may be supported by academic or research institutions, scholarly societies, or commercial interests, or they may charge author fees. Several open-access publishers (BioMed Central, Public Library of Science) charge author fees and also offer memberships to academic institutions, whereby author fees for researchers at the member institution are eliminated or reduced. These membership charges are likely to become unsustainable for library budgets, as they are raised to cover actual costs of publication. Funding agencies may become a primary source of author fees, as they have frequently been for subscription journals' page charges. Researchers can include publication charges in grant proposals, which can take the burden off library budgets and distribute it among societies, foundations, government agencies, and other funding organizations.

A number of large commercial publishers have experimented with a partial open-access model for some or all of their journals (Springer's Open Choice, Blackwell's Online Open, Oxford University Press's Oxford Open, and Elsevier's new Sponsored Articles option), by offering authors the option of releasing their accepted articles immediately upon publication, after payment of a publication fee. Thus, some commercial subscription journal issues now contain both open and restricted articles. Oxford began their experiment

> ...in August 2003, with the announcement of the *Nucleic Acids Research* Open Access experiment. Since then we have extended our experimentation to include a full Open Access model for the whole of *NAR*, an optional Open Access model for *Journal of Experimental Botany*, and full Open Access for the newly-launched journal *Evidence based Complementary and Alternative Medicine (eCAM)*.[19]

It also appears that some authors do not trust that the peer-review process for freely available journals is as rigorous as that for established print journals.[20] Perhaps authors confuse open-access scholarly publishing with self-publishing on the Web. However, the Kauffman-Wills ALPSP study found that all open-access journal publishers surveyed were peer-reviewed except for one review journal.[14] *Nature* started a Web debate about peer review, accompanied by a new model for open review.

> In *Nature*'s peer review trial, lasting for three months, authors can choose to have their submissions posted on a preprint server for open comments, in parallel with the conventional peer review process. Anyone in the field may then post comments, provided they are prepared to identify themselves. Once the usual confidential peer review process is complete, the public "open peer review" process will be closed.[21]

It will be interesting to see the results of this experiment, which is similar to what arXiv[17] has been doing for 15 years. Another perception is that paying an author fee is tantamount to paying to be published. Springer, Oxford, Elsevier, and Blackwell sites indicate that authors may choose to pay for their article to be open access, but they can do so only after the article goes through the acceptance process. This effectively separates the acceptance of an article from the willingness to pay. Public Library of Science (PLoS) offers a waiver in case of need, which is also separate from the editorial and review processes.

CONNECTION BETWEEN JOURNAL PRICING AND OPEN ACCESS

Scholarly open-access publishing offers access to research findings beyond that purchased with subscriptions and thus helps to stretch library dollars. Will researchers take advantage of these new ways of publishing? Faculty authors have the conflicting desire to publish in journals with the highest status or impact, yet want to have their research made widely available. Open-access titles, with a few exceptions, have not yet built their reputations. *PLoS Biology* is a notable exception, as it has an impact factor of 14.672, the highest in the *ISI Journal Citation Reports* biology category. Several BioMed Central titles also ranked among the top five in their categories. As for the wide distribution of research, a recent study appearing in *PLoS Biology* found that open-access articles were cited significantly more frequently than subscription articles from the same journal.[22] This should provide some incentive to authors who might otherwise hesitate to submit their work to open-access journals.

Will including selected articles as open access affect subscription prices? This question about the optional open-access model has been answered in theory by Elsevier for *Nuclear Physics A*, one of their first titles to use their sponsored article option. "When calculating subscription prices we plan to only take into account content published under the subscription model. We do not plan to charge subscribers for author sponsored content."[23] Similar statements appear on the Blackwell, Oxford, and Springer Web sites. It remains to be seen how this will be accomplished, as selected open access is complex to manage on the publisher side and difficult to understand on the library side.

CONCLUSION

It is not known how or whether further developments in open-access publishing will affect journal subscription prices. Although the Directory of Open Access Journals (DOAJ)[24] lists over 2,000 peer-reviewed electronic journals, it appears that in most cases these journals have not been viewed as strong enough competition to cause commercial publishers to lower subscription journal prices.

Will publishers continue to increase subscription prices from 8% to 10% annually? Will libraries cancel subscriptions to important titles and package deals to make it clear to publishers that they cannot support spiraling prices? Will authors flock to open-access journals or open-access choices when available, anticipating higher readership for their research output? Will publishers discover that funding agencies will pay author fees on behalf of researchers and will that become a viable model to support scholarly journal publishing?

These are only a few of the questions raised by the shift to electronic distribution of the journal literature. There are no obvious answers to these questions, but all players–researcher/authors (content providers), publishers (content distributors), librarians (content distribution facilitators), and researchers/readers (content consumers)–have a stake in the outcome. Authors hope for the increased impact of their scholarly research, which can now be distributed openly and widely; commercial publishers and others who are involved in the distribution of scholarly content try to add value in order to make a reasonable profit; librarians anticipate that open-access publishing may provide needed relief to library budgets from the seemingly inexorable rise in journal prices while facilitating the scholarly communication process; and readers simply want to freely read what they find useful for their work. Perhaps these results are not mutually exclusive, and each of the players in this scholarly publication endeavor can reach his or her goal.

REFERENCES

1. Schlimgen, J.B., and Kronenfeld, M.R. "Update on Inflation of Journal Prices: Brandon/Hill List Journals and the Scientific, Technical, and Medical Publishing Market." *Journal of the Medical Library Association* 92, no. 3 (2004): 307-14. Available: <http://www.pubmedcentral.nih.gov/picrender.fcgi?artid=442172&blobtype=pdf>. Accessed: July 20, 2006.

2. Van Orsdel, L.C., and Born, K. "Journals in the Time of Google: Periodicals Price Survey 2006." *Library Journal* 131(April 15, 2006): 39-44. Available: <http://www.libraryjournal.com/article/CA6321722.html>. Accessed: June 14, 2006.

3. Chan, L. "Electronic Journals and Academic Libraries." *Library Hi Tech* 17, no. 1 (1999): 10-6.

4. Tenopir C., and King, D.W. "Towards Electronic Journals: Realities for Scientists, Librarians, and Publishers." *Psycoloquy* 11, no. 84 (2000). Available: <http://psycprints. ecs.soton.ac.uk/archive/00000084/#html>. Accessed: May 31, 2006.

5. Suber, P. "Timeline of the Open Access Movement." Available: <http://www. earlham.edu/~peters/fos/timeline.htm>. Accessed: May 31, 2006.

6. Keyhani, A. "The Online Journal of Current Clinical Trials: An Innovation in Electronic Journal Publishing." *Database* 16(February 1993): 14-23.

7. Berners-Lee, T. "The World Wide Web: A Very Short Personal History." Available: <http://www.w3.org/People/Berners-Lee/ShortHistory.html>. Accessed: June 13, 2006.

8. Tenopir, C. "Online Scholarly Journals: How Many?" *Library Journal* 129 (February 1, 2004). Available: <http://www.libraryjournal.com/article/CA374956.html>. Accessed: June 9, 2006.

9. Cox, J., and Cox, L. *Scholarly Publishing Practice: Academic Journal Publishers' Policies and Practices in Online Publishing.* 2nd ed. Worthing, West Sussex, U.K.: Association of Learned and Professional Society Publishers, 2006. Executive summary available: <http://www.alpsp.org/publications/SPP2summary.pdf>. Accessed: June 13, 2006.

10. Wittig, G.R. "Dual Pricing of Periodicals." *College & Research Libraries* 38, no. 5 (1977): 412-8.

11. Hillson, S.B.; Knight, N.H.; and Newsome, N. "Turning Our World Upside Down: Will Technology Change Pricing?" *NASIG 1998 Proceedings–Workshop 12.* Available: <http://nasig.org/proceedings/1998/workshops/98proc_workshop12.html>. Accessed: June 13, 2006.

12. Siar, J.; Schaffner, M.; and Hahn, K.L. "Proliferating Pricing Models." *Serials Librarian* 48, nos. 1/2 (2005): 199-213.

13. Hitchcock, S.; Carr, L.; and Hall, W. "A Survey of STM Online Journals 1990-95: The Calm Before the Storm." Available: <http://www.cindoc.csic.es/ cybermetrics/pdf/294.pdf>. Accessed: May 31, 2006.

14. Kaufman-Wills Group, LLC. *The Facts about Open Access: A Study of the Financial and Non-Financial Effects of Alternative Business Models for Scholarly Journals.* Worthing, West Sussex, U.K.: Association of Learned and Professional Society Publishers, 2005, p. 1. Available: <http://www.alpsp.org/publications/FAOAcomplete REV. pdf.>. Accessed: May 31, 2006.

15. Cox, J. "Pricing Electronic Information: A Snapshot of New Serials Pricing Models." *Serials Review* 28, no. 3 (2002): 171-5.

16. Arms, W. *Digital Libraries.* Cambridge, MA: MIT Press, 2000, p. 280. Available: <http://www.cs.cornell.edu/wya/DigLib/MS1999/glossary.html>. Accessed: July 17, 2006.

17. arXiv e-print archive. Available: <http://lanl.arxiv.org/>. Accessed: June 13, 2006.

18. Willinsky, J. *The Access Principle: The Case for Open Access to Research and Scholarship.* Cambridge, MA: MIT Press, 2006, p. 212-3. Available: <http://mitpress. mit.edu/books/willinsky/0262232421app1.pdf>. Accessed: June 14, 2006.

19. Oxford Journals. Oxford Open. Available: <http://www.oxfordjournals.org/ oxfordopen/>. Accessed: June 16, 2006.

20. Rowlands, I., and Nicholas, D. "Scholarly Communication in the Digital Environment: The 2005 Survey of Journal Author Behaviour and Attitudes." *Aslib Proceedings* 57, no. 6 (2005): 481-97.

21. Peer Review Trial. Available: <http://www.nature.com/nature/peerreview/index.html>. Accessed: June 15, 2006.

22. Eysenbach, G. "Citation Advantage of Open Access Articles." *PLoS Biology* 4(May 2006): e157. doi: 10.1371/journal.pbio.0040157. Available: <http://biology.plosjournals.org/perlserv/?request=get-document&doi=10.1371/journal.pbio.0040157>. Accessed: June 14, 2006.

23. *Nuclear Physics A*. Available: <http://www.elsevier.com/wps/find/authorshome.authors/nuclearphysicsa>. Accessed: June 14, 2006.

24. Directory of Open Access Journals. Available: <http://www.doaj.org/>. Accessed: July 28, 2006.

doi:10.1300/J383v04n01_03

Extending Electronic Resource Licenses to a Newly Established Overseas Medical School Branch

Michael A. Wood
Carole Thompson
Kristine M. Alpi

SUMMARY. Weill Cornell Medical College in Qatar (WCMC-Q) was established in 2001. This case study describes the establishment and maintenance of access to licensed electronic resources from the libraries of Weill Cornell Medical College in New York City (WCMC-NY) and its parent institution, Cornell University in Ithaca, New York to the new and primarily digital WCMC-Q Distributed eLibrary (DeLib) in Doha, Qatar. Challenges in extending access included defining relationships in a way that vendors could understand, creating networks and support mechanisms on both sides, and communicating across logistical and cultural differences. Through collaboration and coordination, these separately

---

Michael A. Wood, BA, MLS (mawood@med.cornell.edu) is Qatar Liaison Librarian and Assistant Head of Collection Development; Kristine M. Alpi, MLS, MPH (kma2002@med.cornell.edu) is Associate Library Director; both at Weill Cornell Medical Library, 1300 York Avenue, New York, NY 10021. Carole Thompson, MLIS, MBA (cat2004@qatar-med.cornell.edu) is Associate Director, Planning and Digital Initiatives, at Distributed eLibrary, Weill Cornell Medical College in Qatar, P. O. Box 24144, Doha, Qatar.

[Haworth co-indexing entry note]: "Extending Electronic Resource Licenses to a Newly Established Overseas Medical School Branch." Wood, Michael A., Carole Thompson, and Kristine M. Alpi. Co-published simultaneously in the *Journal of Electronic Resources in Medical Libraries* (The Haworth Information Press, an imprint of The Haworth Press, Inc.) Vol. 4, No. 1/2, 2007, pp. 25-40; and: *Electronic Resources in Medical Libraries: Issues and Solutions* (ed: Elizabeth Connor, and M. Sandra Wood) The Haworth Information Press, an imprint of The Haworth Press, Inc., 2007, pp. 25-40. Single or multiple copies of this article are available for a fee from The Haworth Document Delivery Service [1-800-HAWORTH, 9:00 a.m. - 5:00 p.m. (EST). E-mail address: docdelivery@haworthpress.com].

Available online at http://jerml.haworthpress.com
doi:10.1300/J383v04n01_04

25

funded libraries acquire and maintain access to electronic resources at a shared cost. doi:10.1300/J383v04n01_04 *[Article copies available for a fee from The Haworth Document Delivery Service: 1-800-HAWORTH. E-mail address: <docdelivery@haworthpress.com> Website: <http://www.HaworthPress.com> © 2007 by The Haworth Press, Inc. All rights reserved.]*

KEYWORDS. Licensing, remote access, collection development, digital libraries, electronic resources

INTRODUCTION

On April 9, 2001, Weill Cornell Medical College in Qatar (WCMC-Q) <http://www.qatar-med.cornell.edu/> was established when Cornell University <http://www.cornell.edu/>, located in Ithaca, New York, signed an agreement with the Qatar Foundation for Education, Science and Community Development <http://www.qf.edu.qa/> to bring a branch of its medical school to Qatar, which is located in the Middle East region. WCMC-Q is the first American medical school located outside of the United States and is part of a group of university branches opened in Education City, Qatar, near the capital of Doha, that brought an array of higher education to the region.

WCMC-Q maintains the same standards for admission as the Weill Cornell Medical College in New York City (WCMC-NY). WCMC-Q offers both an undergraduate pre-medical and a graduate medical program with separate admission, but reporting to a single Dean. The two-year, non-degree pre-medical program opened in fall 2002, the four-year medical program opened September 2004, and the first M.D. degrees will be granted in 2008.[1-2]

This case report describes the process of extending access to electronic resources licensed by the libraries of WCMC-NY and Cornell University in Ithaca to the new branch in Qatar. Comparisons are made with the case of the Touro University-Nevada experience previously reported by library director Doris Wisher.[3]

Throughout this article, the following abbreviations/acronyms for names and locations are used interchangeably:

- WCMC-Q is the same as Weill Cornell Medical College in Qatar; Qatar branch

- WCMC-NY is the same as Weill Cornell Medical College (New York City); New York City campus
- DeLib is the same as Distributed Electronic Library (Digital library of WCMC-Q)
- CUL is the same as Cornell University Libraries (Ithaca, New York); Ithaca campus

DEFINING THE RELATIONSHIP AMONG BRANCHES

WCMC-Q provides a complete medical education program leading to a Cornell University M.D. degree. The six-year integrated program, consisting of the two-year pre-medical program followed by the four-year medical program, is taught by Cornell faculty. Academic standards are consistent with those of Cornell University in Ithaca and its Weill Medical College in the United States. The pre-medical program consists of courses in the sciences basic to medicine, writing seminars, and medical ethics. In the second year, there is greater emphasis on areas of study that are closer to medicine, such as biochemistry, genetics, and neuroscience. The medical program replicates the curriculum taught at Weill Cornell Medical College in New York City.[4]

Faculty who teach in the WCMC-Q pre-medical program hold Cornell University appointments from the main campus in Ithaca. They are supported by teaching assistants, who are recent Cornell University graduates. WCMC-Q medical program faculty members primarily hold appointments in academic departments at WCMC-NY. A proportion of the faculty resides in Qatar, where they lecture, facilitate small group sessions, counsel, and guide the students. Some faculty members based in New York visit WCMC-Q to deliver teaching modules once they have finished most, or all, of their teaching in New York. In addition, selected lectures are brought to WCMC-Q by streaming video from WCMC-NY and the Ithaca campus. These are normally followed by question-and-answer sessions with the lecturer by interactive videoconferencing.[4] As of academic year 2005-2006, the total number of students for both the pre-medical and medical program exceeds 130 while the total faculty exceeds 40. A comparative profile of both WCMC-Q and WCMC-NY is shown in Figure 1.

FIGURE 1. WCMC-Q and WCMC-NY Profile

Campus	Location	Founded	No. of Faculty	Enrollment 2005-2006
Weill Cornell Medical College in Qatar	Doha, Qatar	2001	Pre-medical–24 Medical–21 Medical-Voluntary–19 Medical-Visiting–12	Class of 2008 (2nd year medical)–16 Class of 2009 (1st year medical)–18 2nd year pre-medical–40 1st year pre-medical–58
Weill Cornell Medical College in New York	New York City, NY	1898	Medical–1,100 (including graduate school faculty)	Class of 2008 (2nd year medical)–100 Class of 2009 (1st year medical)–100 3rd and 4th year medical (combined)–200 Graduate (MA/PhD)–390

DEFINING THE RELATIONSHIP AMONG LIBRARIES

WCMC-NY Library is a physical library with extensive digital collections, on-site computing, and a Web presence. Forty staff members work in the following program areas: access services, administration, cataloging, collection development, computer services, and information services. WCMC-NY Library is one of the many libraries that comprise the Cornell University Libraries (CUL) system. WCMC-NY Library works closely with Cornell University Libraries staff based in Ithaca, particularly those involved in administration, collection development, and technical services. While the Cornell University Libraries have virtual library content, the bulk of the collections is maintained in physical libraries.

In Qatar, the Distributed *e*Library (DeLib) is accessed via more than 100 computers placed in offices, classrooms, labs, and clusters ("pods") throughout the medical branch building and accessible through wired and wireless networks. DeLib gives access to the online information resources of WCMC-Q, WCMC-NY, and Cornell University. At WCMC-Q, handheld computing is emphasized and all medical faculty and first-year medical students are provided with wireless Palm OS Tungsten C personal digital assistants (PDAs). A variety of fee-based and free PDA versions of reference texts, calculators, guides, and evidence-based medicine-related applications provide real-time access in classroom and tutorial learning groups.[5] DeLib also has a single reading room housing a small collection of cataloged print resources. Print is only purchased when electronic versions are not available. Owing to the WCMC-Q Dean's vision of a Roving Reference Team, there is no central reference desk. Librarians follow the flow of information downstream to the desktop and the bench, offering assistance to students and faculty where they work: offices, the pods, the classrooms, seminar rooms, and the labs.[6]

Balancing Independence and Interdependence

WCMC-Q DeLib is an independent library with its own director, library staff, and budget. However, there is frequent communication and the directors of the WCMC-NY and WCMC-Q libraries use video iChat to meet every two weeks. In 2003, the directors agreed on a cost-sharing strategy and formula for extending electronic resource subscriptions from New York to Qatar. During the second half of 2003, they decided that a separate liaison librarian position based in New York was required to assist the head of collection development in New York City in facilitating collaboration and coordination of electronic resources among Qatar, Ithaca, and the New York City locations. Funded by DeLib, the position was established as the Qatar Liaison Librarian and Assistant Head of Collection Development. The liaison librarian started in May 2004 with the primary responsibility of dealing with issues related to delivering electronic resource access to both WCMC-Q and WCMC-NY users. The need for a new position is not unusual; recruitment of an electronic resources librarian also took place at the Touro University-Nevada when they extended virtual access to their new campus.[3]

Timing and personal connections were important as access needed to be established prior to the first class of medical students starting in September 2004. The liaison librarian's first several months were spent working with vendors to add access for the WCMC-Q branch onto medical resource licenses held by the WCMC-NY Library. Working with personnel at CUL Ithaca to add IP ranges onto relevant licenses for the sciences and humanities was crucial for the pre-medical program. In October 2004, the liaison librarian spent a month in Qatar in order to establish personal relationships with DeLib staff and to better understand the needs of the librarians and users. Further relationship development occurred through staff exchanges in efforts to better understand the nature of operations at each library. Library staff connect regularly, from daily communication tools such as phone calls, e-mail messages, and posting, to library staff discussion lists, instant messaging, regular videoconferences, and occasional get-togethers at professional meetings.

During WCMC-Q library's third year of operation, the WCMC-Q library director established a more formal structure. Reference librarians, acting in the role of selectors, formed a collection development team, with one reference librarian chosen as coordinator. An acquisitions support staff person, WCMC-Q library director, and manager of the information services team at WCMC-Q worked principally through the acquisitions and collection coordinators to communicate their needs in terms of acquiring new resources and resolving access issues. The collection coordinator then relayed those needs to the head of collection development and the liaison librarian at WCMC-NY. Processes and procedures change less frequently as more resources are organized and documented, and pass from discovery, selection, and acquisition into a maintenance phase. Further evolution in the collection development process is expected during the clinically-focused third and fourth years of the medical school.

Developing Networks and Support Systems

Creating shared access to resources is further challenged by multiple locations. Many of the CUL Ithaca licenses already included terms to allow or extend access to other campuses regardless of geographic location, which made these resources the easiest to extend. Selection of which resources to adopt first began with links from the CUL Gateway including its catalog <http://www.library.cornell.edu/>. The next resources were Tri-Cat (WCMC-NY library's online catalog), electronic journals, and electronic resources Web pages. All these resources can be accessed from WCMC-NY Library's home page <http://library.med.cornell.edu/>. Tri-Cat is a shared catalog of print and electronic materials from the libraries of Rockefeller University, Memorial-Sloan Kettering Cancer Center, Weill Cornell Medical College, and the Hospital for Special Surgery, and includes thousands of items, primarily print, not accessible by the Qatar branch. The librarians at WCMC-Q wanted to provide access to DeLib resources <http://delib.qatar-med.cornell.edu/> as soon as possible, in order to create their own digital library presence and assist their local users. Due to the difference between the content in Tri-Cat in New York City and the small number of items truly available in Qatar, the WCMC-Q branch acquired its own separate Innovative Interfaces Millennium catalog in July 2003.

Successful provision of seamless access to electronic resources depends a great deal on the capability of the network. To quickly support the educational needs of the pre-medical program to access electronic resources available on the Ithaca campus after WCMC-Q moved from its temporary location on the Qatar University campus into their own permanent building, the Qatar branch IP range was initially subsumed within that of WCMC-NY. Therefore, all access to licensed resources was immediately available without specific negotiation with vendors. However, several months prior to the opening of the first medical class, the WCMC-Q branch acquired its own domain and IP range in order to effectively and efficiently manage its own network in its own time zone and thereby provide more stability and reduce reliance on WCMC-NY. This meant that the liaison librarian needed to work with vendors and the Ithaca campus to get the WCMC-Q branch's new IP range added to the various electronic resource licenses before the medical school term began.

IDENTIFYING AND SELECTING E-RESOURCES

Cornell University Libraries offer a diverse and extensive menu of electronic resources, but not all of the available resources are pertinent to the programs at WCMC-Q. Since the number of full-time equivalent (FTE) students at both the New York City and Qatar locations are very small in comparison (see Figure 1) to FTE at the Ithaca campus, CUL can often include New York City and Qatar in their license agreements for a pro-rated cost or at no additional cost at all. Some of the resources identified, reviewed, and selected from the Ithaca collections include e-books, e-journals, databases, and Web sites. Examples include Knovel, NetLibrary, JSTOR, ProQuest, Biography Index, Dissertation Abstracts, Applied Science and Technology Index, BioOne, LexisNexis, PsycINFO, and RefWorks.

The WCMC-NY campus maintains many unique and separate resources in support of the medical curriculum apart from the Ithaca main campus. Because the FTE of the Ithaca campus is far greater than that of the New York City campus, WCMC-NY generally cannot afford to extend access to its resources to the entire Cornell University community. However, since the Qatar branch duplicates the New York City campus in terms of curriculum, it requires access to the same library resources. This meant extending access to all the resources to which the WCMC-Q campus had licenses either independently or in other arrangements.

Independently-selected resources at WCMC-NY include resources such as Books@Ovid, Journals@Ovid, various databases through Ovid, UpToDate, STAT!Ref, AccessMedicine, MICROMEDEX, MD Consult, and DXplain.

The WCMC-Q collection development team expended a tremendous effort in identifying, vetting, and prioritizing the most desirable resources. The reviewing and selection process began in the online catalogs of both the Ithaca and WCMC-NY campuses. WCMC-Q librarians visited the Cornell University Library Gateway <http://www.library.cornell.edu/> where resources are categorized by subject areas or alphabetically by title. The reference librarian serving as collection coordinator selected additional relevant science resources with the assistance of all reference librarians who selected resources for subject areas and forwarded recommendations. Within each subject area, resources are listed alphabetically with a link to descriptive information and access rights which indicated Cornell community or open access (free). Access rights to the Cornell community did not indicate if access was restricted to any specific Cornell campus. The level of access information and details on permitted usage were generally not sufficient, leaving much for further investigation. Once a resource was reviewed by the WCMC-Q librarian and deemed relevant based on its description, an attempt was made to access that resource. Then further investigation was undertaken to ascertain by whom and where the license was negotiated and held. The WCMC-Q collection coordinator liaised with the WCMC-NY head of collection development and the liaison librarian. Later in the process, the Ithaca campus acquired and installed an Electronic Resources Management (ERM) system from Innovative Interfaces, which in the near future will provide librarians with detailed access rights information from the systematic review of CUL electronic resource licenses. WCMC-Q DeLib has also purchased Innovative's ERM system to better track this information in the future. Access to all the acceptable resources, whether initially accessible or not, was formalized with the licensing library.

LICENSE REVIEW AND NEGOTIATION PROCESS

Selection of resources was a major collaborative effort, but the license review process could only be undertaken by the library holding the license. After the e-resources were reviewed and selected, the license agreements held at the Ithaca and New York City campuses were reviewed to see if they already contained terms that allowed access to branches or multiple sites and to further determine whether to contact the provider to clarify the terms and/or negotiate for expanded access. The head of collection development at WCMC-NY, along with colleagues at CUL, reviewed and re-negotiated license agreements for full-text packages and abstract/indexing databases (some with full or selective full text) through major publishers, vendors, and aggregators as needed. The liaison librarian examined terms of access for single journal titles published by associations and societies without specific license agreements on file.

Contacting Providers of Full-Text Packages and Databases

The head of collection development at WCMC-NY contacted the providers of electronic resources such as Ovid, MD Consult, MICRO-MEDEX, STAT!Ref, AccessMedicine, and UpToDate to request the addition of the new WCMC-Q branch IP range. In some cases, extending access required the signing of a new site license or amending the license with an addendum outlining the site's geographic location and size (FTE). In other instances, some providers charged for adding the WCMC-Q IP range. Other resources that were priced by simultaneous users did not require any changes in the license other than adding the WCMC-Q IP range. For resources that were licensed for a single user or seat, an additional cost was incurred if the WCMC-Q added additional user seats. For example, the WCMC-NY license for Books@Ovid is for access per single user. A single user for the WCMC-Q branch was generally sufficient given the time difference between WCMC-Q and WCMC-NY. However, there were specific titles for which the WCMC-Q wanted the number of users increased. In those cases, WCMC-Q pays a larger share of the cost for these additional seats. There are also a number of resources that WCMC-NY gets access to via Cornell University's membership in the Northeast Research Libraries (NERL) consortium. These resources include Elsevier ScienceDirect, Blackwell Synergy, SpringerLink, and Wiley. The publishers of these resources currently allow the Ithaca, Geneva, and the New York City campuses (including the WCMC-Q branch) to be considered a single site. However, some providers have refused to issue a single cross-campus license, regardless of pricing. While CUL and WCMC-NY license negotiators attempt to find unique solutions, they generally must decide based on what the licensor offers. Expanding access to these resources was a multilayered effort involving a number of parties and extensive time to achieve.

Contacting Associations, Societies, and Small Publishers

WCMC-NY electronic journal collections feature many titles from societies and small publishers that include online access to a number of paid print subscriptions. The liaison librarian contacted these providers as their primarily clinical content was needed for the opening of WCMC-Q's first medical class in September 2004. The majority of these journals were hosted by HighWire Press, and the terms of access described on the journal Web sites restricted access to a single site. For example, the following statements below were taken from the American Association for Clinical Chemistry's "Frequently Asked Questions" Web page for its journal *Clinical Chemistry*.[7] Most of the society publications featured similar statements on their e-journal sites. (Please note: emphasis was added by authors.)

Who from my institution can access *Clinical Chemistry Online*?

An online subscription permits unlimited simultaneous Internet access to *Clinical Chemistry Online* by authorized users generally at one location (the employees, faculty, staff, and students officially associated with the subscriber, and authorized patrons of the subscriber's library facilities that are administered from the subscriber's site or campus) through the use of the institution's IP address. Authenticated and authorized users may access *Clinical Chemistry Online* from other locations (e.g., through dial-in, telnet, etc.).[7]

What is an Institution?

Institutional Online Subscriptions generally provide access to *Clinical Chemistry Online* from an institution in one geographic location and do not permit remote campuses, remote sites, consortia, or other forms of subscription sharing. For the most part, an Institutional Online Subscription authorizes use at a localized site. A "site" is an organizational unit, and may be academic or nonacademic. For organizations located in more than one city, each city office is considered a different site. For organizations within the same city that are administered independently, each office is considered a different site.[7]

For example, each campus in the State University of New York system is considered a different site, and each branch or office of Upjohn Laboratories is considered a different site.[7]

To get beyond this boilerplate, it was necessary to reach out to all the providers. The WCMC-NY liaison librarian compiled a list of all the e-journal titles and publishers with contact information. E-mail was the primary means of contact in order to maintain a paper trail that would serve as an official reference as the formal agreement established and accepted by both parties, since in most cases there was no written license agreement required by the societies, associations, and/or publishers. The liaison librarian and the head of collection development in New York jointly drafted a letter (see Figure 2) that was sent to each of the publishers. In some cases, the responses came back within 24 hours, while others required follow-up e-mails and identifying additional contacts. As a last resort, some publishers were contacted by phone. A variety of responses came back from the societies, associations, and small publishers. Some gave approval to add the WCMC-Q branch IP range at

FIGURE 2. Sample Letter to HighWire Press Publisher

From: Michael Wood [mailto:mawood@med.cornell.edu]
Sent: Friday, July 02, 2004 3:47 PM
To: Customer Services Inquires
Subject: Multiple site access inquiry

Hello AACC Subscription Office

The Weill Cornell Medical Library currently subscribes to the AACC journal "Clinical Chemistry" in print, with online access through HighWire Press.

The Weill Cornell Medical College is starting a new medical school [branch] in Doha, Qatar. The first-year medical students will start this September. There will be approximately 25 students, with around 15 full-time medical faculty. We would like our Qatar [branch] to also have access to our online journals.

Almost all publishers using HighWire Press use this definition of a site:
"For the most part, an institutional subscription authorizes use of the online journal at a localized site." It is the phrase "for the most part" that prompts this inquiry. Would it be possible to add our small Qatar [branch] to our existing license? If not, would it be possible to start a multi-site license with an additional payment that would include online-only access for them? The Qatar library is small, with no room for storing journals, mail delivery is sporadic at best, and they only require online access.

Please let me know at your earliest convenience. Thank you.

Michael Wood
Qatar Liaison Librarian &
Assistant Head of Collection Development
Weill Cornell Medical College Library
1300 York Avenue, C-115
New York, NY 10021
email: mawood@med.cornell.edu
Phone: 212-746-6071

no additional cost due to the fact this was a start-up program with a small FTE. In other responses, FTE was not a factor; the fact that it was a separate branch as per the providers' definition of a site/campus required an additional charge. Some de-identified responses from societies/associations are outlined in Figure 3.

PROMOTING AND MAINTAINING ACCESS

Cataloging Resources

After arrangements were made with content providers, the focus turned to promoting access to the resources through the WCMC-Q's online catalog, a primary access point for the branch users. To populate the catalog, DeLib staff initially loaded bibliographic records from Tri-Cat representing electronic books and journals with available online access in Qatar. The cataloging librarian at WCMC-Q loaded these MARC records with field 856 access links. The initial set of 2,500 + records duplicated from the Tri-Cat had been originally created for print journal titles with electronic access links. These records were not technically accurate for DeLib, as no print collection existed and access was electronic only. Correcting the MARC records to reflect the true state of the primarily

FIGURE 3. De-Identified Publisher Responses to Request to Add WCMC-Q to Existing License

- Under the scenario that you present, we are happy to let you add the Qatar library to your existing license. Should the facility grow and become much larger, I would like to consider adding a separate online site license for them.
- Currently we offer "single" print and online subscriptions to the ABC, and according to this policy you could purchase an additional institutional subscription for your smaller Qatar campus for the time being.
- Our marketing folks will have a proposal for you on Thursday.
- We don't currently have the multiple site license that you are looking for. And with an institutional subscription, access is definitely limited to a single site. As mentioned in the earlier email to your colleague, we are working on different models for licensing for ABC online, but they won't be in place until at least 2006.
- Thank you for your enquiry below. Could you let me know the numbers of academic staff and students on the Qatar campus, and a broad indication of their spread of subject interests in relation to the life sciences and XYZ in particular? We will then get back to you with the proposed terms for any extended access
- We are only able to give access to the ABC online to one site per subscription. If your Qatar campus requires online access they will need to pay for an additional subscription. Thank you.

electronic collection held in WCMC-Q was a project of several months performed by the cataloger with some assistance from paraprofessional staff. Over the first two years, this process of transferring duplicated records was replaced by copy cataloging electronic resource records directly from OCLC and other sources.

When new free or fee-based resources are acquired and access has been extended to the WCMC-Q branch, the liaison librarian informs the WCMC-Q acquisitions coordinator, cataloger, and collection coordinator. The collection coordinator approves the additions to the WCMC-Q catalog and other systems. Upon receiving approval, the WCMC-Q cataloger accesses both the Ithaca and WCMC-NY online catalogs simultaneously via Z39.50 to temporarily copy the bibliographic record in order to facilitate quick access for users until an appropriate, permanent bibliographic record can be obtained.

Solving Access Issues

The impact of the increased number of users on resource access is minimized by the fact that the branches are 6,690 miles apart with a time difference of eight hours (seven hours during daylight savings time in New York). While most users at one location are sleeping, the others have full access. This is especially important for those resources, primarily electronic books, which are limited in terms of simultaneous users or seats. At present, the Qatar branch curriculum, which is identical to the one taught in New York City, follows two weeks behind, further reducing the need for simultaneous use of the same resources.

Despite the stated benefit, the geographic divide creates challenges. One downside of relying on shared access is the lack of local control. Since licenses are negotiated and held by the Ithaca and New York City campuses, when users at the Qatar branch occasionally experience access failure, these issues must be brought to the attention of the liaison librarian for resolution via appropriate channels. Due to time and schedule differences, problem solvers and liaison staff at the WCMC-NY and Ithaca campus libraries or vendor offices are most likely not at work and blissfully unaware of urgent issues faced by a presenting instructor or student doing last-minute research in Qatar. The culture of Qatar is reflected in the modified workweek of Sunday through Thursday, leaving only four shared working days. This can complicate scheduling and contact with the Ithaca and New York City campuses and U.S.-based vendors. Currently, DeLib staff forwards all access inquiries to the acquisitions coordinator, who e-mails the liaison librarian with a copy to the head of collection development at WCMC-NY. No data are available on the frequency of access problems; anecdotally, the number of e-mails received has decreased over time. Access-related problems, such as the prompting for username and password, continued for several months after the change of WCMC-Q IP addresses until the resource providers implemented the changes.

Usage of Electronic and Print Resources

Many electronic resources provide statistics on online use. However, it has been difficult to divide usage by the Ithaca campus, New York City campus, and the Qatar branch as most publishers/vendors provide statistics only for the total IP range and do not make it possible to break them out more specifically. Statistics for the Qatar branch have been an ongoing concern due to the need to document justifications for all types of spending for the branch. This problem is not unique to this case study; clearly, innovation in the area of usage statistics for collaboratively-purchased resources is needed.

There are resources that the WCMC-Q branch cannot access electronically because of license restrictions or the lack of a subscription to the electronic format at either the Ithaca or New York City campus. To facilitate access to these electronic or print resources available on a Cornell campus, DeLib staff send an interlibrary loan (ILL) request via e-mail, fax, Ariel, or ILLiad to the holding library, where the document is faxed or digitized and sent back to the WCMC-Q within 24 hours. For resources not held by a Cornell library, WCMC-NY Library provides interlibrary loan and document delivery service to the WCMC-Q users. Requests are made through the ILLiad direct request system. While the electronic access to DeLib was being established and stabilized via the WCMC-Q network and IP range, a fair amount of ILL traffic was received by WCMC-NY. Between July 2004 and June 2005, 320 requests were filled by WCMC-NY and other U.S. libraries. Since the start of the second-year medical class, activity is stable with 318 requests made to WCMC-NY from July 2005 to June 2006. In addition, DeLib staff use ILLiad to order and obtain full text from the document delivery systems of CISTI or the British Library.

Continued Coordinated Collection Development

As current practice, collection development is a coordinated effort between the head of collection development at the WCMC-NY campus and the collection coordinator librarian at the Qatar branch. Costs of electronic resources are primarily shared on a 50/50 basis. However, in cases in which staff at one branch wish to increase the number of simultaneous users but staff at another branch feel that there will be little use, the added cost is paid by the branch that made the proposal. When staff at one library suspect there to be little interest in a resource, a different cost-sharing model is negotiated between New York City campus and Qatar branch. WCMC-Q contacts CUL in Ithaca to join in licenses for resources that are out of scope for the WCMC-NY campus, but that are needed for the undergraduate pre-medical curriculum. Resources considered necessary for the Qatar medical and pre-medical programs or other site-specific needs may be selected and acquired directly by Qatar. Examples of resources that Qatar purchased directly are Reuters Health News, which provides health news for the DeLib Web site, and the Gold Standard Suite, which has been installed on PDAs issued on the WCMC-Q campus.[5]

CONCLUSION

The major benefit of extending electronic resource access to the WCMC-Q branch is that cost sharing resulted in a significant increase in purchasing power for both libraries. Similarly, Wisher reported that group purchasing resulted in savings of approximately 50% in the book and journal budget for the Touro University-Nevada virtual library.[3] Now that access to resources has been established, there are new questions to be answered about interlibrary loan and document delivery provisions, access to online resources through portal sites, and the impact of federated searching on use of licensed resources. WCMC-Q and WCMC-NY library staff regularly converse on these and other issues such as online reserve materials and the use of PDA resources that will require changes in practice.

Times have changed. When this project was first initiated, few publishers were open to, or offering, multi-site or enterprise-wide licensing of electronic resources. Now that more enterprise-wide licensing is becoming available, it will be necessary to revisit the licenses in future years. CUL has formed a task force that will look into the issues and problems relating to cross-campus access to electronic resources as collaborative programs and research expand across Cornell campuses. The workforce and workflow in libraries are also changing to better address the demands of electronic resource management. In 2005, CUL reorganized distributed technical services operations to create an over-arching library technical services unit which includes sections related to acquisitions and cataloguing, and e-resources and serials management. A PDF version of the CUL Technical Services organizational chart can be found on the Web.[8] Working through the selection, access, promotion, and maintenance of electronic resources in collaboration with the Ithaca campus's new structure will provide new opportunities for the librarians at WCMC-NY and WCMC-Q to enhance electronic resource access for library users wherever they may be.

REFERENCES

1. Cornell University. Qatar Campus. Available:<http://en.wikipedia.org/wiki/Weill_Cornell_Medical_College_in_Qatar>. Accessed: June 9, 2006.

2. Weill Cornell Medical College in Qatar. Available: <http://www.qatar-med.cornell.edu/aboutUs/index.html>. Accessed: June 9, 2006.

3. Wisher, D. "The Touro University-Nevada Virtual Library." *Journal of Electronic Resources in Medical Libraries* 2, no. 3(2005): 1-12.

4. Cornell University. Qatar Campus. Available: <http://www.cornell.edu/visiting/qatar/>. Accessed: June 1, 2006.

5. Joc, K., and Thompson, C. "Application and Usage of Wireless PDAs in a First-Year Medical Curriculum." *Journal of Electronic Resources in Medical Libraries* 3, no. 1 (2006): 89-94.

6. "Roving Reference: Service 'In Context.'" Available: <http://www.qatar-med.cornell.edu/mediaNews/reports/2004/rovingref.html>. Accessed: June 9, 2006.

7. Clinical Chemistry. Frequently Asked Questions about Institutional Subscriptions. Available: <http://www.clinchem.org/subscriptions/institutional-faq.shtml>. Accessed: June 9, 2006.

8. Cornell University. Technical Services Organizational Chart. Available: <http://www.library.cornell.edu/tsweb/deptinfo/orgcharts.pdf>. Accessed: June 9, 2006.

doi:10.1300/J383v04n01_04

Access to Health Information
in Latin America and the Caribbean

C. Verônica Abdala
Rosane Taruhn

SUMMARY. This article provides an overview of the initiatives to improve access to health information in Latin America and the Caribbean regions, particularly cooperative activities developed through the Virtual Health Library (VHL) of the Latin American and Caribbean Center on Health Sciences Information (BIREME). VHL's Portal of Journals has facilitated access to scientific journals and increased usage by integrating content available through Scientific Electronic Library Online (SciELO) and Health InterNetwork Access to Research Initiative (HINARI). The authors relate BIREME networking efforts and other actions to the high percentage of HINARI logins from Latin America and Caribbean countries. doi:10.1300/J383v04n01_05 *[Article copies available for a fee from The Haworth Document Delivery Service: 1-800-HAWORTH. E-mail address: <docdelivery@haworthpress.com> Website: <http://www. HaworthPress.com> © 2007 by The Haworth Press, Inc. All rights reserved.]*

C. Verônica Abdala, MA (veronica.abdala@bireme.org) is Manager of Cooperative Information Services, and Rosane Taruhn (taruhnro@bireme.ops-oms.org) is Librarian Consultant, both for Latin American and Caribbean Center on Health Sciences Information/Pan American Health Organization/World Health Organization, Rua Botucatu, 866, São Paulo, Brazil 04023-901.

[Haworth co-indexing entry note]: "Access to Health Information in Latin America and the Caribbean." Abdala, C. Verônica, and Rosane Taruhn. Co-published simultaneously in the *Journal of Electronic Resources in Medical Libraries* (The Haworth Information Press, an imprint of The Haworth Press, Inc.) Vol. 4, No. 1/2, 2007, pp. 41-50; and: *Electronic Resources in Medical Libraries: Issues and Solutions* (ed: Elizabeth Connor, and M. Sandra Wood) The Haworth Information Press, an imprint of The Haworth Press, Inc., 2007, pp. 41-50. Single or multiple copies of this article are available for a fee from The Haworth Document Delivery Service [1-800-HAWORTH, 9:00 a.m. - 5:00 p.m. (EST). E-mail address: docdelivery@haworthpress.com].

Available online at http://jerml.haworthpress.com
© 2007 by The Haworth Press, Inc. All rights reserved.
doi:10.1300/J383v04n01_05

KEYWORDS. E-journals, electronic journals, health information, developing countries, BIREME, Virtual Health Library, SciELO, HINARI, PAHO, Latin America, Caribbean region

INTRODUCTION

Different initiatives that promote the use of health information worldwide[1] underscore the importance of information access to education and health care research. Many of these initiatives are driven by inequities in accessing information and knowledge, mainly in developing countries, despite the proliferation of electronic information resources. In this context, librarians have long faced difficulties providing access to their users.

In Latin America and the Caribbean region, this situation is aggravated by the libraries' limited budgets, which results in the lack of information and human resources. This article offers a perspective on how such limitations were overcome through the establishment in 1967 of a cooperative network between the Pan American Health Organization (PAHO) and Latin America and Caribbean countries. This effort is unique because of its ongoing operation and coverage of nearly all countries in the region.

This network's startup date coincides with the creation of *Biblioteca Regional de Medicina* (BIREME), the Spanish term for regional medical library. Though still called BIREME, its name was changed in 1982 to Latin American and Caribbean Center on Health Sciences Information to better express its evolution from a classical library paradigm toward an information center and to better reflect the expansion of subjects covered ranging from biomedical information to the entire field of health sciences.

The network set the priority of controlling the literature created in the regions through the production of Latin American and Caribbean Literature on Health Science Information (LILACS) database. LILACS is still considered an essential bibliographic resource that complements access to international literature contained in the MEDLINE database.

The development of these cooperative and network-based efforts were in response to the strategic guidelines defined by PAHO and the World Health Organization (WHO) to promote access to relevant information products and services.[2] Currently BIREME promotes, coordinates, and operates three major networks within the region that focus on universal access to information and knowledge:

- VHL–Virtual Health Library <http://www.bvsalud.org> is a common space that is becoming the standard resource for accessing, publishing, and evaluating health sciences information and knowledge in Latin America and Caribbean countries.
- SciELO–Scientific Electronic Library Online <http://www.scielo.org> is a model for cooperative electronic publishing of scientific journals on the Internet especially conceived to meet the communication needs of Latin America and the Caribbean. It provides an efficient way of assuring universal visibility and accessibility to its scientific literature, overcoming the phenomenon known as "lost science."
- ScienTI–International Network of Information and Knowledge Sources to Support Science, Technology and Innovation <http://www.scienti.net> is a regional network of councils, institutions, and research groups oriented to the development of methodological and technological solutions for the management of research directories, projects, and institutions.

ACCESS TO JOURNALS THROUGH VHL

During different stages of BIREME's history, the organization has promoted cooperative efforts to provide access to journals in Latin America. In 1969, BIREME defined the creation of a collective catalog of scientific journals as one of its priorities, complemented by the exchange and donation of materials among libraries.

Since then, this catalog has played a critical role in the operation of regional interlibrary loan services, through the Cooperative Service for Accessing Documents (SCAD). SCAD allows shared use of the libraries' collections and cooperates with the VHL Network to fill over 300,000 document requests per year from users in the regions.[3]

VHL's Portal of Journals on Health Sciences is the outcome of the cooperative collection development work. Portal of Journals is a catalog with metadata, bibliographic descriptions (title, ISSN, publisher, etc.), and availability and access mode information for print and electronic titles. It operates as a facilitating central access point to e-journals, including those titles promoted by SciELO, HINARI, CAPES Portal, and other open access initiatives.

Until May 2006, VHL's Portal of Journals gathered metadata from more than 13,000 scientific journals, including full-text access information and corresponding links for almost 5,000 titles. Over 7,700 journals are available in the holdings of 82 cooperating libraries.[3]

SciELO–Scientific Electronic Library Online

SciELO <http://www.scielo.org/> is a joint effort, which started in the 1990s, intended to disseminate electronic access and provide visibility to scientific journals in Latin America and the Caribbean region. As of July 2006, SciELO offered its users free online access to 289 full-text scientific journals from Brazil, Chile, Cuba, Venezuela, and Spain. The number of journals is constantly growing and other countries (Argentina, Colombia, Costa Rica, Mexico, Peru, Uruguay, and Portugal) are developing their SciELO collections.

CAPES Periodicals Portal

"Programa Periódicos CAPES" <http://www.periodicos.capes.gov.br> is a program of the Brazilian government that offers electronic access to more than 9,000 international and national journals and to 90 databases in all areas of knowledge for more than 170 Brazilian educational institutions. The use of this portal is free of charge for users affiliated with participating Brazilian institutions.

HINARI in Latin America and the Caribbean Region

The Health InterNetwork Access to Research Initiative (HINARI) <http://www.who.int/hinari/en/> provides free or very low-priced online access to the major journals in biomedical and related social sciences fields to local, non-profit institutions in developing countries. The HINARI program, set up by WHO together with major publishers, enables developing countries to gain access to one of the world's largest collections of biomedical and health literature.

HINARI was launched in January 2002, after several meetings and discussions with six major publishers (Blackwell, Elsevier Science, Harcourt Worldwide STM Group, Wolters Kluwer International Health & Science, Springer Verlag, and John Wiley) about the financial difficulties faced by poor countries interested in subscribing to international journals. Latin American countries contributed to this effort by recommending "shared access to scientific e-journals" during the 2nd Regional Coordination Meeting of the VHL, held in Havana, Cuba in April 2001:

...We shall make a special appeal to the WHO, the leading international organization on health, and its partners, to contribute to the efforts conducted domestically and internationally in order to:

- Liaise with governments urging them to take on an active role to support and provide information services on health;
- Negotiate with the private sector, including commercial publishers as well as IT and communication providers, so that they commit to offer fair prices, within the reach of all interested parties, and build an infrastructure capable of reaching out to the excluded communities.
- Support initiatives aiming at providing free access to scientific literature.[4]

Eligibility

HINARI initially allowed non-profit institutions in countries with a gross national product (GNP) per capita of less than US$1,000 a year to receive free online access to more than 1,500 journal titles. In 2003, the initiative expanded eligibility to allow institutions in countries with a GNP per capita between $1,000 and $3,000 per year to access online material available through HINARI. In 2006, the number of publishers involved in HINARI increased to 70, providing access to more than 3,300 journals and other text resources.

Health and medical institutions can join the initiative by filling out an online form. After processing and authenticating the submitted information, WHO staff issue a password to the institution. The HINARI Web portal provides free access to full-text biomedical and related social sciences articles supplied by the publishers involved in the initiative. The portal also allows users to conduct PubMed literature searches and search for journals by subject.

The numbers of participating publishers, journals, and other full-text resources has grown continually. More than 1,100 institutions in 113 countries, distributed throughout six regions–Eastern Mediterranean (EMRO), Europe (EURO), South-East Asia (SEAR), Africa (AFRO), America (AMRO), and Western Pacific (WPRO)–now access HINARI. Figure 1 shows the distribution of institutions registered in HINARI, by region, and the total number of registered institutions with active access by June 2005.[4]

FIGURE 1. Distribution of HINARI Institutions by Region

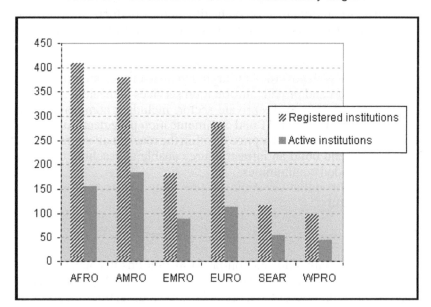

In the American Region (AMRO), including the Caribbean, 19 countries have benefited from the HINARI initiative:

(a) Phase I (free access): Guyana, Haiti, Honduras, and Nicaragua
(b) Phase II (low-cost access): Belize, Bolivia, Colombia, Costa Rica, Cuba, Dominican Republic, Ecuador, El Salvador, Guatemala, Jamaica, Panama, Paraguay, Peru, Suriname, St. Vincent, and the Grenadines

In 2005 alone, HINARI registered roughly 1,800,000 logins from institutions in 104 countries throughout the six regions. The vast majority (65%) of logins came from AMRO (America & Caribbean Regions).[5] Figure 2 breaks down the 2005 distribution of HINARI logins by region.

According to Aronson,[6] usage depends more on Internet connectivity than the economic wealth of the country, as some very low-income countries, such as Ethiopia, are among HINARI's biggest users. The high cost of reliable Internet access has limited the expansion of services. HINARI cannot reach everyone who might benefit. In many

FIGURE 2. Distribution of HINARI Logins by Region

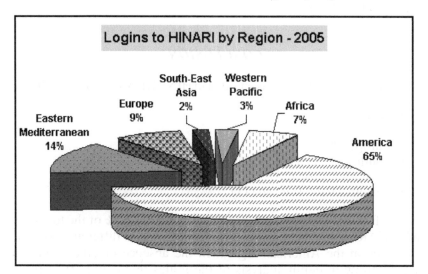

countries, Internet access is slow, expensive, and unreliable. HINARI provides access to 3,300 journals:

> [h]owever, some valuable journals of specific relevance to the developing world (tropical medicine journals, for example) may not be available through HINARI as this may compromise the publishers' commercial viability. In addition, in some countries, publishers withhold some journals because their sales are significant in these countries.[7]

This is the case in Colombia, Peru, and some other Latin American countries. But even so, Peru and Colombia are the two countries recording the largest number of HINARI logins.

Despite these problems with withheld journals, in Latin America and the Caribbean region, networking activities and promotion of free access to HINARI journals have resulted in effective use and expanded access to health information. BIREME carried out different promotional activities to libraries including conducting workshops, using VHL Portal of Journals to provide integrated access to e-journals, and translating Web site content into Spanish and Portuguese languages. These actions have significantly boosted the number of HINARI logins from institutions located in Latin America and the Caribbean to 65% of the total number of logins.

CONCLUSION

Distribution of institutions enrolled in HINARI by region is as follows:

- Africa (36)
- America (18)
- Europe (20)
- South-East Asia (6)
- Western Pacific (13)
- Eastern Mediterranean (11)

The fact that the American region accounts for 65% of the total sum of HINARI logins begs the question as to what is different about the countries in the American region. In the absence of other data that would allow in-depth analysis of the issues that could affect these figures, much credit to such results must be given to cooperative networking efforts consolidated in Latin America and the Caribbean region and materialized by the ongoing development of the Virtual Health Library.

Since its establishment, BIREME has contributed significantly to the region's capacity to access health sciences-related information, knowledge sources, and systems. BIREME continues to promote cooperative work in the region but cannot replace its responsibilities to organize and lead network actions to promote access to health information. This subject has been widely discussed during the VHL network technical meetings as reflected in the policy document featured in the Appendix of this article.

VHL, SciELO, CAPES Portal, HINARI, and other initiatives that provide access to health information are not alone sufficient to promote information usage; they are solely the "raw material" to be processed and disseminated. In order to maximize results, these initiatives should continue, and governments and institutions should develop policies and provide funding. In addition, libraries should broaden their service capacities, make services more efficient, and explore opportunities to participate in an organized and cooperative network environment such as the VHL.

REFERENCES

1. Zaher, C.R., and Packer, A.L. "O desenvolvimento da informaçâo em Saúde na América Latina e Caribe e perspectivas futures." *Ciência da Informação 22*, no. 3 (1993): 193-200.

2. World Health Organization. *Knowledge Management. Knowledge Management Strategies*. Available: <http://www.who.int/kms>. Accessed: July 5, 2006.

3. BIREME (Latin America and Caribbean Center on Health Sciences Information). *Relatório para o Comitê Assessor Nacional do Convênio de Manutenção da BIREME*. I Reunião do ano 2006. Soã Paulo: BIREME, 2006.

4. Conclusiones y recomendaciones. Grupa 7. Acceso compartido a las revistas científicas electrónicas. Available: <http://crics5.bvsalud.org/E/grupos/grupo7/conclusao. htm>. Accessed: September 12, 2006.

5. World Health Organization. *HINARI Login Indicators by Region, Countries, and Institutions*. Internal document, June, 2005.

6. Aronson, B. "Improving Online Access to Medical Information in Low-Income Countries." *New England Journal of Medicine 350*(March 4, 2004): 966-8.

7. Katikireddi, S.V. "HINARI: Bridging the Global Information Divide." *BMJ 328*(May 15, 2004): 1190-3. Available: <http://bmj.bmjjournals.com/cgi/content/full/ 328/7449/1190>. Accessed: July 3, 2006.

doi:10.1300/J383v04n01_05

APPENDIX

Policy Proposal to Expand the Access to Health Scientific Journals in Latin America and Caribbean Regions

Considering that the equitable access to information in health sciences is fundamental for the improvement in life conditions of the region's population, the Internet and particularly the VHL–Virtual Health Library–that may have the potential of transform this goal into a reality, both national and international institutions are called on to support this initiative and contribute to:

1. cooperative development of journals collections in the VHL

   • with the main focus on the users' information needs
   • with the objective of reducing title duplications and costs
   • with the purpose of increasing the number of titles with collection in the Collective Catalog SeCS–(Serials Catalog in Health Sciences), available at the Journals Portal <http://portal-revistas.bvs.br/>

2. formalization of national initiatives regarding cooperative services such as interlibrary loan and development of collective catalogs for shared access to collections, both in paper and electronic formats.
3. configuration of consortia at the national level aiming at the electronic access to selected groups of international journals, with accessible prices for developing countries.
4. incentive to use journals' free access programs.
5. participation, dissemination, and incentives for using Information Access Programs to electronic Journals, such as the following:

   • HINARI program for eligible countries according to criteria
   • Brazil's CAPES Periodicals Program for participating institutions

6. encouragement of publication of electronic journals in the region
7. qualifying of users for the health information access services

Note: This proposal is a continuation of the conclusions and recommendations made by Working Group 7. Shared Access to Electronic Journals during the 5th Regional Conference on Health Sciences Information (CRICS 5) <http://crics5.bvsalud.org/E/grupos/grupo7/conclusao.htm> held in Havana, Cuba from April 25-27, 2001.

Assessing Online Use:
Are Statistics from Web-Based Online
Journal Lists Representative?

Rick Ralston

SUMMARY. Many library Web sites feature hypertext lists of their online journals. This article explores the reliability of usage statistics generated by these Web-based journal lists. Reliability is assessed by comparing the number of journal title accesses from the list with the number of articles downloaded per title supplied by electronic journal vendors. The study includes 468 titles from three different vendors. While a correlation in use from the two different sources was found, this sample's usage counts from the online journal list were not accurate enough to use with cancellation decisions. doi:10.1300/J383v04n01_06 *[Article copies available for a fee from The Haworth Document Delivery Service: 1-800-HAWORTH. E-mail address: <docdelivery@haworthpress.com> Website: <http://www. HaworthPress.com> © 2007 by The Haworth Press, Inc. All rights reserved.]*

KEYWORDS. Collection development, electronic journals, usage statistics

Rick Ralston, MSLS (rralston@iupui.edu) is Assistant Director for Library Operations, Ruth Lilly Medical Library, Indiana University School of Medicine, 975 W. Walnut Street, Indianapolis, IN 46202.

[Haworth co-indexing entry note]: "Assessing Online Use: Are Statistics from Web-Based Online Journal Lists Representative?" Ralston, Rick. Co-published simultaneously in the *Journal of Electronic Resources in Medical Libraries* (The Haworth Information Press, an imprint of The Haworth Press, Inc.) Vol. 4, No. 1/2, 2007, pp. 51-64; and: *Electronic Resources in Medical Libraries: Issues and Solutions* (ed: Elizabeth Connor, and M. Sandra Wood) The Haworth Information Press, an imprint of The Haworth Press, Inc., 2007, pp. 51-64. Single or multiple copies of this article are available for a fee from The Haworth Document Delivery Service [1-800-HAWORTH, 9:00 a.m. - 5:00 p.m. (EST). E-mail address: docdelivery@haworthpress.com].

doi:10.1300/J383v04n01_06

INTRODUCTION

Librarians have an urgent need to make informed decisions regarding journal subscriptions. This is not a new necessity, but the library environment has changed drastically with the meteoric rise in user preference for electronic journals over print journals.[1] What collection managers most want to know about their journal subscriptions is if they are being used and if the level of use justifies the cost. They would also like to know who is using them and how. Librarians were fairly comfortable with methods of assessing the use of print journal collections and used these to base their cancellation decisions.[2] However, when the new online environment gave publishers and aggregators responsibility for hosting library journal collections, new ways of assessing usage had to be devised.[3]

A complicating factor in devising these new usage assessment methods is the rapidly changing nature of the technology used to make online journals available. Whereas in the early years librarians struggled to make electronic journals easily accessible,[4] there are now often a multiplicity of ways to access full-text journal content. Another factor inhibiting the ability to assess usage has been the inconsistency or lack of vendor-provided statistics. Thankfully, this situation has changed rapidly over the last few years. Many vendors now provide COUNTER-compliant statistics[5] that make it much easier to compare the use of journals from different content providers. It is still not easy to pull statistics together from multiple sources, and there are still a significant number of situations without good usage statistics.

The objective of this study was to determine if cancellation decisions for electronic journal subscriptions could be reliably based on the usage statistics collected from the alphabetical list of electronic journals provided by the Indiana University School of Medicine Libraries' Web site. While these statistics are not as comprehensive as vendor-supplied statistics in that they only record title level accesses rather than the number of articles downloaded, this study was intended to test the hypothesis that usage rank from online journal list statistics correlates with usage rank from vendor-supplied statistics. If this hypothesis proves true, then journal list usage statistics can be used in cancellation decisions.

SETTING

The Indiana University School of Medicine (IUSM) Libraries include the Ruth Lilly Medical Library (RLML), the Center for Bioethics Reference Center, and the Morrison Ophthalmological Library, which are all located on the Indiana University-Purdue University Indianapolis (IUPUI) campus, and the Steven C. Beering Medical Library located at the Northwest Center for Medical Education in Gary, Indiana. The RLML is the main library for the IUSM; it houses the largest medical book and journal collection in the state and includes 270,000 volumes and 1,900 current journal subscriptions. It is the primary information resource for faculty, staff, and students of the Indiana University School of Medicine, School of Nursing, School of Health and Rehabilitation Sciences, and licensed Indiana health care professionals.

The library contracts with a commercial firm to generate and maintain a list of electronic journals on its Web site. This list includes approximately 1,100 titles that the library subscribes to directly as well as about 2,500 titles that are free or are available through consortial agreements. Many titles are available through more than one source, and in these cases a link to each source is provided under the title. Links are also provided for each title from the online catalog record to the corresponding title in the list. OpenURL linking is also available from the library's electronic citation databases to the corresponding full-text articles.

METHODS

This study selected 468 titles from two publishers and one aggregator. These titles represent over 40% of the library's online journal subscriptions. The time period covered by the statistics was calendar year 2004. All current subscriptions from the three vendors that were active for the entire year were included in the study. For the time period covered, the two publishers provided COUNTER-compliant statistics while the aggregator did not. For COUNTER-compliant statistics, the "Number of Successful Full-Text Article Requests by Month and Journal" report was used. For aggregator statistics, the number of full-text views reported for each title was used.

Usage statistics for the online journal list were compiled using a report that shows how many times each source for each title was clicked on. For example, for a title that was accessible to users both through a publisher link and an aggregator link, this report shows a separate count for each source. For this study, only the count from the vendor being compared was used. Using this example, only the number of linkouts from the publisher link for that title in the online journal list was compared to the count for that title provided by the publisher.

Reports from the three vendors and the journal list were compiled in a single spreadsheet showing the number of full-text articles downloaded for each title as reported by the vendor as well as the number of linkouts reported for that title by the journal list. The titles were then ranked from highest to lowest use by both the vendor count and the journal list count. Columns were added for the ratio of the vendor count to the journal list count, and the difference in ranking based on the two different counts and a percentage displacement was calculated by dividing the rank difference by the total number of titles in the list. An excerpt from this table is shown in Table 1.

In order to determine the degree of correlation between the set of paired rankings, the measure of correlation was calculated using the Spearman Rank Correlation Coefficient.[6] A summary of the results by vendor is presented in Table 2. Correlation coefficients range from negative one (−1) to one (1), with negative one being a perfect negative correlation, one being a perfect positive correlation, and 0 being no correlation.

RESULTS

The degree of rank correlation among all titles is illustrated in Figure 1 with a scatter plot. An exact correlation would be represented by all the points in a straight line running from the lower left corner where the highest use titles are represented to the upper right corner where the lowest use titles are represented. While there is a definite correlation between the rank based on use from the journal list and rank based on use from vendor reports, the question remained whether there was enough of a correlation to warrant basing cancellation decisions on the journal list statistics. The number of points plotted high in the upper left quadrant of the graph points out the problem encountered with this method. These are titles with high vendor-reported usage but with low usage according to online journal list statistics. Relying on list statistics for these titles would result in the cancellation of high-use titles.

The degree to which titles were displaced in the list is demonstrated in Figure 2. This pie graph shows that 50% of the titles were displaced from their true position in the list by more than 10%, assuming that the vendor rank represents the true position. To put that in understandable terms, the situation is analogous to being twentieth in line among 467

TABLE 1. Online Journal List Titles with Highest Usage Count

Title	Vendor Use	List Use	Ratio	Vendor Rank	List Rank	Rank Difference	% Displacement
JAMA: Journal of the American Medical Association	11,517	2009	5.73	1	1	0	0.00%
New England Journal of Medicine	7,470	1767	4.23	3	2	1	0.21%
Nature	1,931	1059	1.82	34	3	31	6.62%
Neurology	2,970	916	3.24	17	4	13	2.78%
AACN Clinical Issues	1,654	879	1.88	46	5	41	8.76%
Journal of the American College of Cardiology	3,856	696	5.54	8	6	2	0.43%
Cancer	1,728	679	2.54	41	7	34	7.26%
Critical Care Medicine	3,244	632	5.13	12	8	4	0.85%
Circulation	2,449	628	3.90	23	9	14	2.99%
American Journal of Cardiology	2,525	624	4.05	21	10	11	2.35%

TABLE 2. Online Journal Usage Comparison

	Titles	Average Vendor Use	List Use	Ratio	Rank Correlation
Aggregator	267	814	126	6.47	0.67
Publisher 1	149	699	132	5.29	0.84
Publisher 2	52	396	123	3.21	0.84
All	468	731	128	5.73	0.72

$P < 0.000001$ for all correlations in this table.

FIGURE 1. Correlation of Usage Rank from Online Journal List and Vendor Reports

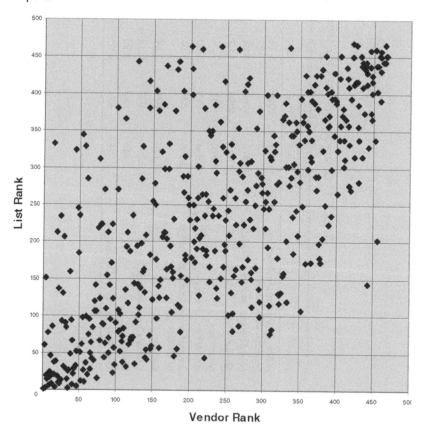

FIGURE 2. Percentage Displacement of Journals in Ranked List

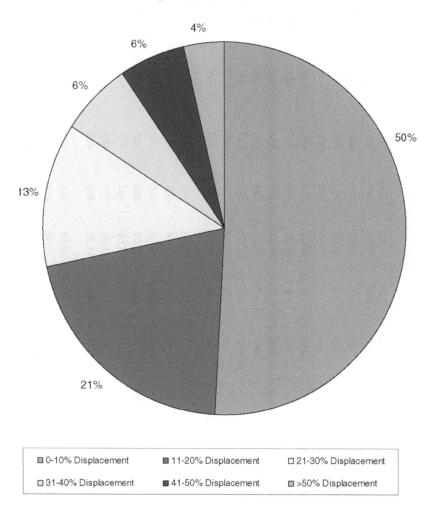

people waiting at the Bureau of Motor Vehicles and being told to move to sixty-seventh in line.

To simulate a subscription cancellation situation, the bottom 10% of the online journal list titles was selected for cancellation as shown in Tables 3 and 4. Titles that would not have been canceled according to vendor usage statistics are shown in boldface type. Out of 47 titles selected

TABLE 3. Bottom 10% of Titles Based on Online Journal List Usage Statistics, Part 1

Title	Vendor Use	List Use	Ratio	Vendor Rank	List Rank	Rank Difference	% Displacement
Inside Case Management	**101**	**4**	**25.25**	**421**	**468**	**-47**	**-10.04%**
Journal of Clinical Engineering	23	5	4.60	465	466	-1	-0.21%
Milbank Quarterly	88	5	17.60	426	466	-40	-8.55%
Family and Community Health	**394**	**6**	**65.67**	**242**	**464**	**-222**	**-47.44%**
Health Care Manager	**496**	**6**	**82.67**	**201**	**464**	**-263**	**-56.20%**
Topics in Emergency Medicine	**220**	**7**	**31.43**	**336**	**463**	**-127**	**-27.14%**
Implant Dentistry	**342**	**8**	**42.75**	**266**	**460**	**-194**	**-41.45%**
Journal of Endodontics	**461**	**8**	**57.63**	**216**	**460**	**-244**	**-52.14%**
Texas Heart Institute Journal	51	8	6.38	452	460	-8	-1.71%
International Journal of Gynecological Pathology	62	9	6.89	445	459	-14	-2.99%
Point of Care	37	10	3.70	460	458	2	0.43%
Biomedical Safety and Standards	13	11	1.18	468	452	16	3.42%
Birth Defects Research Part B	44	11	4.00	458	452	6	1.28%
Journal of Head Trauma Rehabilitation	**147**	**11**	**13.36**	**385**	**452**	**-67**	**-14.32%**
Journal of Thoracic Imaging	78	11	7.09	432	452	-20	-4.27%
Obstetric Anesthesia Digest	20	11	1.82	467	452	15	3.21%
Topics in Health Information Management	**125**	**11**	**11.36**	**405**	**452**	**-47**	**-10.04%**
Diagnostic Molecular Pathology	43	12	3.58	459	450	9	1.92%
Topics in Clinical Nutrition	101	12	8.42	421	450	-29	-6.20%
Birth	**752**	**13**	**57.85**	**129**	**443**	**-314**	**-67.09%**

TABLE 4. Bottom 10% of Titles Based on Online Journal List Usage Statistics, Part 2

Title	Vendor Use	List Use	Ratio	Vendor Rank	List Rank	Rank Difference	% Displacement
Dermatology Nursing / Dermatology Nurses' Association	**548**	**13**	**42.15**	**184**	**443**	**-259**	**-55.34%**
Evidence Based Dentistry	33	13	2.54	463	443	20	4.27%
Evidence-Based Eye Care	26	13	2.00	464	443	21	4.49%
Journal of Cardiovascular Risk	71	13	5.46	435	443	-8	-1.71%
Journal of Nutritional Biochemistry	68	13	5.23	439	443	-4	-0.85%
Neurosurgery Quarterly	23	13	1.77	465	443	22	4.70%
Clinical Dysmorphology	76	14	5.43	433	439	-6	-1.28%
Clinical Neurology and Neurosurgery	68	14	4.86	439	439	0	0.00%
Problems in General Surgery	50	14	3.57	454	439	15	3.21%
Ultrasound Quarterly	46	14	3.29	456	439	17	3.63%
Artificial Intelligence in Medicine	62	15	4.13	445	437	8	1.71%
Orthopaedic Nursing	**590**	**15**	**39.33**	**168**	**437**	**-269**	**-57.48%**
ASAIO Journal	**115**	**16**	**7.19**	**413**	**436**	**-23**	**-4.91%**
Addictive Disorders and Their Treatment	**155**	**17**	**9.12**	**380**	**433**	**-53**	**-11.32%**
Lippincott's Case Management	**493**	**17**	**29.00**	**202**	**433**	**-231**	**-49.36%**
Survey of Anesthesiology	69	17	4.06	438	433	5	1.07%
Critical Care Nursing Quarterly	**558**	**18**	**31.00**	**182**	**432**	**-250**	**-53.42%**
Clinical Imaging	66	19	3.47	441	429	12	2.56%
Current Opinion in Otolaryngology and Head and Neck Surgery	**133**	**19**	**7.00**	**396**	**429**	**-33**	**-7.05%**
Journal of Clinical Apheresis	37	19	1.95	460	431	29	6.20%
Current Opinion in Endocrinology and Diabetes	57	20	2.85	448	425	23	4.91%
International Anesthesiology Clinics	**185**	**20**	**9.25**	**357**	**425**	**-68**	**-14.53%**
Matrix Biology	**167**	**20**	**8.35**	**371**	**425**	**-54**	**-11.54%**
Topics in Magnetic Resonance Imaging	**158**	**20**	**7.90**	**377**	**425**	**-48**	**-10.26%**
Cancer Cytopathology	113	21	5.38	414	422	-8	-1.71%
Oral Microbiology and Immunology	128	21	6.10	403	422	-19	-4.06%
Tobacco Control	**314**	**21**	**14.95**	**280**	**422**	**-142**	**-30.34%**

for cancellation, 22 were not in the bottom 10% according to vendor statistics and of those 22, seven titles ranked in the top half according to vendor statistics. This exercise verified the problem identified in the scatter plot: the correlation breaks down at the low use end of the online journal list statistics, precisely where it is needed to make accurate cancellation decisions.

DISCUSSION

An analysis of the 22 titles revealed that all but two were from the aggregator and disproportionately represented nursing titles. This suggests that users of the aggregated resource are less likely to access these titles from the online journal list than users of titles purchased directly from the publisher, particularly those users searching the nursing literature. This was also predicted in the summary data of Table 2 where the aggregator titles showed less correlation than the publisher titles and a higher ratio of vendor use to list use. This is similar to the result obtained by Wulff and Nixon when comparing the print use of a title to its online use.[7] Their sample showed that the online titles from the aggregator had more use per title and a higher ratio of online to print use than the titles in two publisher packages. The authors speculated that ease of access from the aggregator's citation databases to its full-text journals made those journals more popular with users and accounted for the higher ratio. This same phenomenon may be a factor in this study as well, since there is greater ease in linking from the aggregator's databases to its full-text articles than using the OpenURL links to access journals from other vendors.

It should also be noted that nursing students, many of whom are undergraduates, often use the university library on the IUPUI campus and are not as likely to use the Medical Libraries' online journal list. As shown in Tables 5 and 6, nearly all of the journals with the highest negative rank difference are nursing journals. In Jaguszewski and Stemper's study comparing local online journal list usage and vendor-supplied counts, they hypothesized a "bookmarking effect" where researchers and students in one discipline might be more prone to bypass the online journal list than those in other disciplines.[8] They did not find such an effect in their study, however, which showed that usage statistics from their online journal list were accurate enough to be used in collection development decisions. Bookmarking may be a factor in this study, though. The journals from the aggregator have a higher percentage of

TABLE 5. Titles with Largest Negative Rank Displacement, Part 1

Title	Vendor Use	List Use	Ratio	Vendor Rank	List Rank	Rank Difference	% Displacement
Journal of Cataract and Refractive Surgery	3,107	47	66.11	14	332	-318	-67.95%
Birth	752	13	57.85	129	443	-314	-67.09%
Home Healthcare Nurse	1,559	43	36.26	54	344	-290	-61.97%
Public Health Nursing	1,679	49	34.27	44	324	-280	-59.83%
Nursing Administration Quarterly	927	33	28.09	101	380	-279	-59.62%
Journal of Cardiovascular Nursing	684	22	31.09	144	417	-273	-58.33%
Journal of Emergency Nursing : JEN	1,447	48	30.15	57	328	-271	-57.91%
Orthopaedic Nursing	590	15	39.33	168	437	-269	-57.48%
Health Care Manager	496	6	82.67	201	464	-263	-56.20%
Dermatology Nursing / Dermatology Nurses' Association	548	13	42.15	184	443	-259	-55.34%
Oral Surgery, Oral Medicine, Oral Pathology, Oral Radiology and Endodontics	842	37	22.76	112	366	-254	-54.27%
Critical Care Nursing Quarterly	558	18	31.00	182	432	-250	-53.42%
Nursing Education Perspectives	664	26	25.54	153	403	-250	-53.42%
Journal of Endodontics	461	8	57.63	216	460	-244	-52.14%
Geriatric Nursing (New York, N.Y.)	684	33	20.73	144	380	-236	-50.43%
Journal of Nursing Management	1,195	53	22.55	77	312	-235	-50.21%
Lippincott's Case Management	493	17	29.00	202	433	-231	-49.36%
Clinical Nurse Specialist : CNS	1,434	63	22.76	61	285	-224	-47.86%
Family and Community Health	394	6	65.67	242	464	-222	-47.44%
Journal of Perinatal & Neonatal Nursing	611	32	19.09	164	385	-221	-47.22%
Current Opinion in Psychiatry	655	34	19.26	157	377	-220	-47.01%
Journal of the American Medical Directors Association	521	26	20.04	191	403	-212	-45.30%
Nursing Management	2,390	78	30.64	24	234	-210	-44.87%
Journal of Cardiopulmonary Rehabilitation	565	34	16.62	180	377	-197	-42.09%

TABLE 6. Titles with Largest Negative Rank Displacement, Part 2

Title	Vendor Use	List Use	Ratio	Vendor Rank	List Rank	Rank Difference	% Displacement
Nurse Educator	1,649	75	21.99	48	245	-197	-42.09%
Journal of the American Board of Family Practice	493	28	17.61	202	398	-196	-41.88%
AORN Journal	2,726	84	32.45	19	213	-194	-41.45%
Implant Dentistry	342	8	42.75	266	460	-194	-41.45%
Psychological Medicine	727	48	15.15	136	328	-192	-41.03%
Journal of Nursing Scholarship	1,630	77	21.17	50	236	-186	-39.74%
Mechanisms of Development	1,065	67	15.90	85	270	-185	-39.53%
Journal of Clinical Nursing	2,251	86	26.17	28	207	-179	-38.25%
CIN: Computers, Informatics, Nursing	382	22	17.36	247	417	-170	-36.32%
ANS, Advances in Nursing Science	924	67	13.79	102	270	-168	-35.90%
JONA'S Healthcare Law, Ethics, and Regulation	447	33	13.55	219	380	-161	-34.40%
Gastroenterology Nursing	587	47	12.49	172	332	-160	-34.19%
Journal of Pediatric Nursing	617	51	12.10	162	321	-159	-33.97%
Journal of Infusion Nursing	409	32	12.78	233	385	-152	-32.48%
American Journal of Physical Medicine & Rehabilitation	733	63	11.63	134	285	-151	-32.26%
Nursing Standard	6,634	114	58.19	4	151	-147	-31.41%
Cancer Nursing	1,121	81	13.84	80	223	-143	-30.56%
American Journal of Infection Control	1,120	81	13.83	81	223	-142	-30.34%
Nurse Practitioner	1,201	83	14.47	76	218	-142	-30.34%
Tobacco Control	314	21	14.95	280	422	-142	-30.34%
Journal for Nurses in Staff Development	1,635	101	16.19	49	185	-136	-29.06%
Nuclear Medicine and Biology	324	23	14.09	277	413	-136	-29.06%
Psychosomatic Medicine	602	58	10.38	166	298	-132	-28.21%

nursing titles than the two publisher packages. It should also be noted that Jaguszewski and Stemper's study did not include titles from an aggregator, which appears to be a major cause of the discrepancies in this study.

CONCLUSION

The results of this study do not support reliance on online journal list usage statistics for cancellation decisions unless no other statistics are available. While there is a correlation of rank across the whole list, this correlation is not as strong in subgroups of titles and is particularly weak on the low end of usage counts from the online journal list.

If journal list usage statistics must be used, this study indicates that electronic journals within an aggregator database may have disproportionately low list accesses. One should also look for patterns in the titles with low list use and consider whether users of those titles might have special circumstances that would cause them to bypass the online journal list. Certainly list accesses should not be equated with articles downloaded, as this study found an average ratio of 5.73 articles downloaded for each title access recorded on the list. These results should encourage librarians to insist that electronic journal vendors supply them with COUNTER-compliant usage statistics. Librarians have very little information on which to base collection development decisions without these data.

REFERENCES

1. De Groote, S.L., and Dorsch, J.L. "Online Journals: Impact on Print Usage." *Bulletin of the Medical Library Association* 89, no.4 (2001): 372-8.

2. Ralston, R. "Use of a Relational Database to Manage an Automated Periodical Use Study." *Serials Review* 24, nos.3/4 (1998): 21-32.

3. Luther, J. "White Paper on Electronic Journal Usage Statistics." *Serials Librarian* 41, no.2 (2001): 119-48.

4. Bishop, A.P. "Logins and Bailouts: Measuring Access, Use, and Success in Digital Libraries." *Journal of Electronic Publishing* 4, no. 2 (1998). Available: <http://www.press.umich.edu/jep/04-02/bishop.html>. Accessed: July 17, 2006.

5. COUNTER. "Counter–Online Usage of Electronic Resources." Available: <http://www.projectcounter.org/index.html>. Accessed: July 17, 2006.

6. Wessa, P. "Free Statistics Software." version 1.1.18: Office for Research Development and Education. Available: <http://www.wessa.net/>. Accessed: July 17, 2006.

7. Wulff, J.L., and Nixon, N.D. "Quality Markers and Use of Electronic Journals in an Academic Health Sciences Library." *Journal of the Medical Library Association* 92, no.3 (2004): 315-22.

8. Jaguszewski, J.M., and Stemper, J.A.. "Usage Statistics for Electronic Journals: An Analysis of Local and Vendor Counts." *Collection Management* 28, no. 4 (2003): 3-22.

doi:10.1300/J383v04n01_06

Two Interfaces, One Knowledge Base: The Development of a Combined E-Journal Web Page

Felicia Yeh
Karen McMullen

SUMMARY. Over the past few years, the libraries of the University of South Carolina (USC) have experienced a significant increase in the number of journals added to their electronic collections. As more and more e-journal challenges arose, it became apparent that an e-journal management system was needed to administer the rapidly growing collection. After a thorough selection process, TDNet was selected. The purpose of this article is to describe how two separate libraries within the USC system successfully collaborated in the implementation of a shared electronic journals management system. In early 2003, Thomas Cooper Library, along with the School of Medicine Library, proposed a combined e-journal list. Due to the collective efforts of librarians from both libraries and the e-journal management system vendor, the combined page made its debut to the faculty, staff, and students in early 2004. doi:10.1300/J383v04n01_07 *[Article copies available for a fee from The Haworth Document Delivery Service: 1-800-HAWORTH. E-mail address: <docdelivery@haworthpress.com>*

Felicia Yeh (felicia@gw.med.sc.edu) is Assistant Director for Collections Management, School of Medicine Library, University of South Carolina, 6311 Garners Ferry Road, Columbia, SC 29208. Karen McMullen (karen.mcmullen@sc.edu) is Serials Acquisitions Librarian, Thomas Cooper Library, University of South Carolina, 1322 Greene Street, Columbia, SC 29208.

[Haworth co-indexing entry note]: "Two Interfaces, One Knowledge Base: The Development of a Combined E-Journal Web Page." Yeh, Felicia, and Karen McMullen. Co-published simultaneously in the *Journal of Electronic Resources in Medical Libraries* (The Haworth Information Press, an imprint of The Haworth Press, Inc.) Vol. 4, No. 1/2, 2007, pp. 65-73; and: *Electronic Resources in Medical Libraries: Issues and Solutions* (ed: Elizabeth Connor, and M. Sandra Wood) The Haworth Information Press, an imprint of The Haworth Press, Inc., 2007, pp. 65-73. Single or multiple copies of this article are available for a fee from The Haworth Document Delivery Service [1-800-HAWORTH, 9:00 a.m. - 5:00 p.m. (EST). E-mail address: docdelivery@haworthpress.com].

Available online at http://jerml.haworthpress.com
doi:10.1300/J383v04n01_07

KEYWORDS. Combined Journal Manager, electronic journals, electronic resource management systems, ERM, TDNet

INTRODUCTION

Prior to purchasing TDNet, the University of South Carolina (USC) Thomas Cooper (TC) Library and the School of Medicine (SOM) Library each had its own home-grown e-journal Web page that provided access to their e-journal holdings. With the rapid growth of e-journal titles at both libraries, it quickly became apparent that library staff members were no longer able to maintain links and update titles to the publisher databases on these pages.

After careful evaluation of several e-journal management systems, TDNet e-journal management system was selected and successfully implemented in 2003 for all USC libraries, with the exception of the Law Library. TDNet created one Journal Manager Web page for TC Library, SOM Library, and the seven regional campus libraries. Via the "choose to view per library" box, users can select and browse e-journal holdings by campus; however, access to full-text holdings at other libraries was not permitted. TC and SOM libraries found this limitation to be a major concern because of agreements and commitments to provide cooperative electronic access. The limitation was brought to TDNet's attention and after extensive communication with the two libraries, it was proposed that a combined Journal Manager Web page would give users full-text access to e-journal holdings at both libraries, leaving the seven other USC regional libraries unchanged.

SETTING

USC is a public institution founded in 1801. The university's main campus is located in downtown Columbia, South Carolina with seven regional campuses located throughout the state. The university has more than 35,900 students and approximately 2,000 faculty on the eight campuses. The university's primary mission is to serve the educational needs of the citizens of South Carolina through teaching, research, service, and creative activity.

USC houses seven libraries, including SOM Library, on the main campus in Columbia and seven additional libraries at the regional campuses. The primary mission of the USC libraries is to acquire, organize, and promote the use of scholarly collections supporting the educational, research, and service missions at USC.

Founded in 1974, the USC School of Medicine is located at the Dorn Veterans Affairs Medical Center, which is approximately eight miles from the main USC Columbia campus. The primary mission of the USC School of Medicine is to improve the health of the people of the state of South Carolina through the development and implementation of programs for medical education, research, and the delivery of health care. SOM Library's mission is to provide quality library and information services to support the education, research, and service programs of the School of Medicine, and to provide quality health information to the people of South Carolina.

DEVELOPMENT OF THE COMBINED PAGE

Originally, the TDNet page included individual title listings for nine USC libraries, plus a tenth listing (All Libraries) that combined all the library collections into one list. TDNet outlined two options for the development of a single listing that would show separate entries for TC Library/SOM Library titles:

- Option #1–Create a new library listing on the existing TDNet page

Under this option, TC Library and SOM Library lists would be combined into one separate list on the TDNet existing page thereby providing easier access for users. However, remote user support would be limited because each title could only be listed once. Since the libraries maintain separate proxy servers, it would be necessary to choose between supporting TC Library or SOM Library proxy users. There would also be no library abbreviations such as "USCC" and "USCM" in the title listing.

- Option #2–Develop a separate "satellite" TDNet page

Under this option, a new TDNet page would be set up for these two libraries only. Both sites could link from the main page and the new TC Library/SOM Library page. The advantage of this model was that both libraries would regain the ability to support remote users. A potential drawback of the combined page was the loss of the comprehensive list that features the holdings of the seven regional campus libraries.

After reviewing both options, the libraries strongly favored the second option, which supported remote access (see Figures 1 and 2).

TWO INTERFACES, ONE KNOWLEDGE BASE

In early 2004, the combined page was fully implemented. TDNet hosts two separate Journal Manager Web sites for the USC libraries:

- <http://tdnet.com/scg> is a list of all e-journal holdings for TC Library, SOM Library, and the seven regional campus libraries.
- <http://tdnet.com/usccsom> is a separate Web site that contains the combined e-journal holdings of only the TC Library and SOM Library.

An important criterion was to make sure users were provided with the same holdings information in either TDNet Web site. When changes to online holdings were made, library staff made sure that the changes were reflected in both TDNet Web sites.

TDNet built a connection from the online administrator function in the original Journal Manager Web site to the holdings in the new combined Web site, allowing easy holdings updates (see Figure 3). When holdings are changed in the main administrator function, they are reflected in the main page. The changes are automatically copied in real-time to the combined page, keeping the holdings identical in both Web sites. At the same time, the individual libraries can maintain unique user interfaces and other customization preferences in the separate Web sites.

BENEFITS

The main purpose of creating a combined list was to simplify the searching process for users and library staff looking for online titles. Three major benefits have been identified since the inception of the combined page:

- Users: Users no longer have to look at individual libraries' e-journal title lists. The combined page provides all available access points for e-journals owned by either library. This not only saves time by

FIGURE 1. Combined Page of TC Library and SOM Library

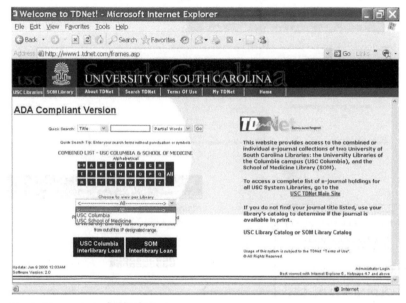

FIGURE 2. Example of Journal Title Search in the Combined Page

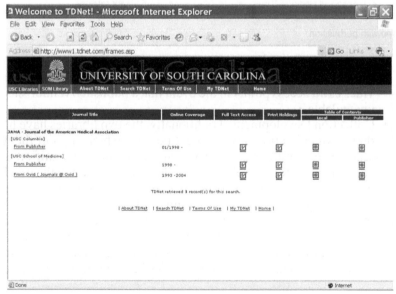

FIGURE 3. Example of the Two Interfaces

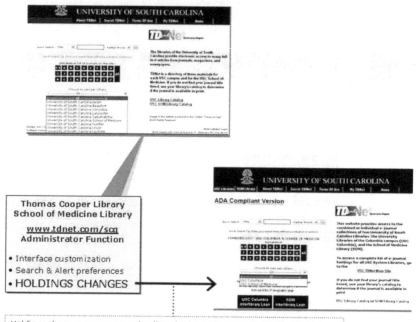

Holdings changes are processed online via the main U.South Carolina TDNet website. Holdings changes are automatically copied to the combined Thomas Cooper & School of Medicine TDNet website in real-time. Each library retains control over the appearance and functionality of the different TDNet websites.

furnishing a centralized location to access e-journal titles, it provides extra access points in the event that a publisher/vendor site is unavailable.

- Collection Development: Traditionally, the two libraries have had their own collection development policies which support the research needs of their users. The combined list has magnified the value of collection development collaboration between the two libraries. Collaborative efforts have been initiated related to purchasing e-journals and eliminating duplicate e-journal titles. In the past two years, the two libraries participated in numerous consortial purchasing initiatives via PASCAL (Partnership Among South Carolina Academic Libraries) and the Carolina Consortium. Access to the number of e-journal titles has significantly increased for users. Both libraries have benefited from resource sharing and cost savings.

- Library Staff: The collaboration between the serials staff in both libraries has reduced the duplicative efforts required for the daily maintenance of the e-journal title list in TDNet. Staff time has decreased significantly related to negotiating with publishers/vendors, activating new titles, updating current titles, solving access problems, maintaining links, and removing titles.

PROBLEMS/ISSUES WITH THE COMBINED PAGE

As new systems are implemented, problems are to be expected. The primary issues faced by the libraries include:

- Communication Issues: Communication between the serials staff of the two libraries was not consistent whenever changes were made to an individual library's holdings. As a result, e-journal pages sometimes displayed inconsistent holdings information.
- Maintenance of Journal Notes: Both libraries are required to maintain their Journal Notes in separate pages. When a journal note is needed, it is necessary for both libraries to input it in their individual pages in order for the note to display on both libraries' pages.
- Training Issues: Training issues involve not only users but library staff as well. Users perceive that the online catalog is a one-stop shop to access all library resources when in fact both libraries do not catalog all e-journals. Library staff, particularly those working in public services areas, need training to educate library users that TDNet should be used as the main access point for e-journals. Library staff need to point users to the combined page in order to access both libraries' e-journal holdings simultaneously. The SOM Library maintains not only the titles to which they subscribe but selectively adds titles that are "biomedical" in nature from aggregators such as ScienceDirect and KluwerOnline as well as links to individual titles held by TC Library. TC Library's policy is to add purchased titles to the catalog and TDNet. For titles that the library has access to, but does not pay for, the titles are only added to TDNet and are not placed in the catalog.

FUTURE IMPROVEMENTS

The problems of the combined page were identified and communicated to the vendor. TDNet proposed to create a separate library list in the current page that would automatically combine the holdings of TC Library and SOM Library (see Figure 4). This change was recommended because it would offer the following advantages:

1. Eliminates the need for a separate TDNet Web site for each library.
2. Journal Notes setup in TC Library or SOM Library will automatically appear in the new combined list, which currently has to be manually repeated in each individual library e-journal page.

FIGURE 4. The Future Look of the Combined Page

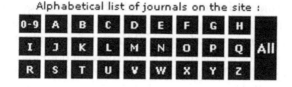

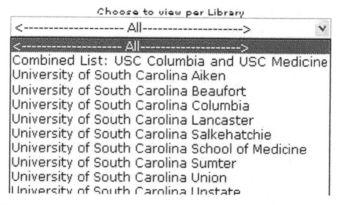

3. The ability to customize the name of the combined list (as it appears in the choose to view per library menu), and to provide a special URL that links directly to the combined title list.

CONCLUSION

The creation of the combined TDNet page has been challenging. With the collective efforts of the two libraries and TDNet, numerous obstacles have been resolved. Library staff and users alike have benefited from the implementation of the combined page. Currently, users accessing the SOM Library page can access 2,741 titles. TC Library page users can access 30,660 titles. Via the combined page, however, the total number of titles will increase to more than 31,000. TDNet has provided tremendous support throughout the implementation process. The two libraries and TDNet will continue to collaborate and are committed to enhancing the combined page for the benefit of their users.

REFERENCES

1. University of South Carolina, Office of Institutional Planning & Assessment. "2005-2006 Mini Fact Book." Available: <http://kudzu.ipr.sc.edu/factbook/2006/>. Accessed: June 4, 2006.

2. University of South Carolina, University Libraries. "Library Overview." Available: <http://www.sc.edu/library/mission.html>. Accessed: June 6, 2006.

3. University of South Carolina, School of Medicine. "University of South Carolina School of Medicine Bulletin." Available: <http://www.sc.edu/bulletin/SOM/SOM.html>. Accessed: June 6, 2006.

4. University of South Carolina, School of Medicine. *Communications, the Newsletter of the School of Medicine Library.* January 2003. Available: <http://uscm.med.sc.edu/com29.htm>. Accessed: August 18, 2006.

doi:10.1300/J383v04n01_07

Off-Campus User Behavior:
Are They Finding Electronic Journals
on Their Own or Still Ordering
Through Document Delivery?

Julie A. Garrison
Pamela A. Grudzien

SUMMARY. This study investigates how off-campus students at Central Michigan University interact with electronic journals in an environment where a full-service document delivery option is available to them. Wiley InterScience and Project MUSE online access statistics are compared with document delivery requests for articles available in these online packages. The study found that increasingly students are accessing the material themselves through the online packages and document delivery requests are decreasing. doi:10.1300/ J383v04n01_08 *[Article copies available for a fee from The Haworth Document Delivery Service: 1-800-HAWORTH. E-mail address: <docdelivery@haworthpress.com> Website: <http://www. HaworthPress.com> © 2007 by The Haworth Press, Inc. All rights reserved.]*

Julie A. Garrison, MLIS (julie.garrison@cmich.edu) is Director of Off-Campus Library Services, and Pamela A. Grudzien, MSL, MSA (grudz1pa@cmich.edu) is Head of Technical Services; both at Central Michigan University, Park Library, Mount Pleasant, MI 48859.

[Haworth co-indexing entry note]: "Off-Campus User Behavior: Are They Finding Electronic Journals on Their Own or Still Ordering Through Document Delivery?" Garrison, Julie A., and Pamela A. Grudzien. Co-published simultaneously in the *Journal of Electronic Resources in Medical Libraries* (The Haworth Information Press, an imprint of The Haworth Press, Inc.) Vol. 4, No. 1/2, 2007, pp. 75-85; and: *Electronic Resources in Medical Libraries: Issues and Solutions* (ed: Elizabeth Connor, and M. Sandra Wood) The Haworth Information Press, an imprint of The Haworth Press, Inc., 2007, pp. 75-85. Single or multiple copies of this article are available for a fee from The Haworth Document Delivery Service [1-800-HAWORTH, 9:00 a.m. - 5:00 p.m. (EST). E-mail address: docdelivery@haworthpress.com].

KEYWORDS. Electronic journals, document delivery, Project MUSE, Wiley InterScience, off-campus students, Web Access Management, usage statistics

INTRODUCTION

Today's complex library environments provide access to electronic journals through a variety of means. Publishers make their journals available through their own interfaces, sold by individual title as well as in package deals. Many of the online subscription databases also provide access to full-text articles online. Library catalogs and citation databases link to online journals through the use of link resolver software. While more full text is increasingly available to users as they conduct online database searches, there is also a sense that it takes a more diligent and savvy library user to understand these different options and successfully retrieve materials by him- or herself. To users who take classes through extended learning, removed from the physical library, navigating the digital library may seem even more perplexing. This study attempts to measure the independence of one off-campus community where "finding it yourself" is not required and mediated document delivery is readily accessible.

BACKGROUND

Since electronic journals have proliferated over the past ten years and the significant portion of library budgets is spent on expanding in this area, libraries have investigated their impact in a number of areas. Studies have measured their effect on interlibrary loan and document delivery services, and have looked at whether expanded e-journal collections result in a decreased number of non-returnable requests, a decrease in interlibrary loan and document delivery staff workload, and lower costs spent in obtaining material.

In 2000, librarians at Ball State University conducted a series of studies that examined the percentage of full-text online articles requested through interlibrary loan that were available through aggregate databases. They found very few borrowing or lending requests could be filled through available databases and concluded that because the results were not significant enough, it was not cost-effective to search the databases before processing requests.[1] Published that same year, a study done at the

University of North Carolina-Chapel Hill concluded it was still difficult to assess the potential of full-text articles to reduce the need for inter-library loan.[2]

A few years later, Glasgow University Library staff studied whether there was a link between "bundled" e-journals and lower document de-livery requests. Document delivery patterns showed a decline of nearly 80% for titles available in their Elsevier package between 1998/1999 and 2001/2002. They also reported that while the number of requests for books remained more stable over the past decade, there has been a significant drop in disposables (photocopied journal articles), indicating there is some correlation between this decline and the increasing avail-ability of full-text electronic journals.[3]

Yue and Syring found that usage of Elsevier online journals increased each year during a four-year study period, between July 1999 and June 2003. Forty-seven percent of these uses were from journals that were also owned in print in the University of Nevada, Reno Library. During this same period, they saw a fluctuation in interlibrary loan workload and requests. Their study noted an increase in the number of canceled interlibrary loan requests for materials owned by the library and sug-gested further analysis of how users interact with their online libraries.[4]

In another review, Echeverria looked at interlibrary loan statistics from various countries which indicated that document delivery demand is re-ducing as electronic journal availability is increasing.[5] The John Jay College of Criminal Justice study reinforced this argument by reporting that their total number of requests has decreased each year since 2000.[6]

All of these studies focused on filling requests for items users consid-ered unavailable at their own institutions, and looking at the interlibrary loan functions of the library. To date, very few studies have discussed the impact of electronic journal availability on document delivery ser-vices, particularly services tailored to fill requests for items known to be owned by the library and available to the university community.

OFF-CAMPUS LIBRARY SERVICES

Central Michigan University's Off-Campus Library Services depart-ment is designed to serve the non-traditional, working student who takes classes remotely through the university's extended degree programs. The majority of students are enrolled in master's level programs, with some in undergraduate or doctoral programs. Services include a guaranteed 24- to 48-hour turnaround time for processing materials owned within the university library and available on the shelf. Students have the option of ordering materials even if the materials are available online to the university community. Therefore, the document delivery service processes and fills requests for items students can retrieve on their own through the digital library.

Student requests can be e-mailed, entered into a Web form, taken by phone via a toll-free telephone number, or submitted via a toll-free fax number. Off-Campus Library Services reference librarians encourage students to take advantage of the document delivery service if they experience any difficulties retrieving materials on their own. Students may also take mediated search results, sent via e-mail from the reference librarians, and forward these directly to the document delivery office for processing without ever logging in to a database themselves. Off-Campus Library Services are included as part of the off-campus tuition and there are no limits on the number of requests a student can make. Because of this "full service" philosophy, there is interest in investigating how often off-campus students take the initiative to find full-text articles online through their own searching as opposed to requesting these items through the document delivery service.

METHODOLOGY

This study looked at two well-known e-journal packages and compared direct online off-campus student access to the document delivery requests made for articles available in these two packages. The two e-journal packages were: Wiley InterScience, a group of journals weighted toward medicine and psychology; and Project MUSE, a collection of journals in the humanities and social sciences. These packages were selected because the subject areas correlated well with two major degree programs offered through Off-Campus Programs: the Master of Administration with a Health Management concentration and the Master of Humanities.

The choice was made to use the library's Innovative Interfaces Web Access Management (WAM) proxy server statistics to estimate the percentage of unmediated access as students are delineated by patron type upon login, making it easy to isolate off-campus student use. One major drawback to using WAM is the statistics are calculated based on every file that goes through the proxy server. Therefore, in addition to the hypertext page, one or more graphic files may also be counted each time a page is loaded. Also, access to a resource through WAM does not necessarily equate with access to a full-text journal article. A student might have authenticated to a resource, but then did not find the needed information or clicked through several pages before finding the actual text of the journal article. In January 2006, Innovative Interfaces changed the way WAM counts, thereby inflating the numbers significantly and making comparisons from the previous year difficult. Given these limitations, statistics were reviewed on a month-by-month basis, comparing off-campus access with overall access to calculate the percentage of off-campus use.

To get a better feel for actual usage, the percentage calculated from the WAM statistics was then multiplied by vendor-supplied data to estimate the number of articles accessed by off-campus students. While these data are not perfect, they provide a more realistic idea of the significance of the WAM numbers. These were calculated and examined on a monthly basis as there was no overall consistency in the WAM statistics when compared to the vendor numbers.

Usage data supplied by both selected vendors was compliant with the COUNTER Code of Practice. COUNTER (*Counting Online Usage of Networked Electronic Resources*) <http://www.projectcounter.org/> is an international coalition of librarians, publishers, and intermediaries that has designed a set of standards and protocols to be used in recording and exchanging online usage data. COUNTER's Code of Practice provides definitions of data elements, guidance on data to be collected and measured, and formats for reporting usage. Since both vendors complied with this COUNTER Code, their statistics on full-text article retrieval were considered valid and reliable for this study.

The document delivery statistics were calculated by pulling specific journal request information from the Clio and ILLiad databases for the study period. Central Michigan University's Document Delivery Office switched to the ILLiad system in February 2006. Because each request is documented, numbers provide accurate off-campus usage. The period of comparison for the Wiley and Project MUSE titles date from the time the packages were turned on for off-campus students in January 2005, providing 1.5 years worth of data (see Table 1).

RESULTS

Wiley InterScience

Dividing the off-campus WAM numbers into the overall WAM figure for Wiley InterScience, it appears that off-campus has made up approximately 9% of usage over the 1.5 year study period. Multiplying the

TABLE 1. Comparison of Online and Document Delivery Requests for Wiley InterScience and Project MUSE

Month	Wiley InterScience			Project MUSE		
	Estimated Online	Document Delivery	Total	Estimated Online	Document Delivery	Total
January 2005	3	88	91	21	12	33
February 2005	0	81	81	4	29	33
March 2005	0	63	63	6	14	20
April 2005	15	48	63	13	19	32
May 2005	11	42	53	2	12	14
June 2005	21	49	70	17	13	30
July 2005	48	35	83	0	25	25
August 2005	29	26	55	15	12	27
September 2005	27	42	69	5	14	19
October 2005	42	65	107	78	23	101
November 2005	10	49	59	67	17	84
December 2005	16	11	27	15	13	28
January 2006	58	66	124	20	18	38
February 2006	52	33	85	13	16	29
March 2006	28	42	70	19	13	32
April 2006	18	36	54	16	8	24
May 2006	79	53	132	3	7	10
June 2006	67	4	71	13	14	27
Total	616	833	1449	226	279	505

calculated monthly percentage of off-campus WAM access with the monthly vendor-supplied data for the database reveals an upward trend (see Table 2). Between January-June 2005 and July-December 2005, there was a 244% increase in online access. From January to June 2006, there was another 76% increase. During the first six months of the study, 12% of off-campus access came from the online resource. This figure increases to 43% in the second six-month period, and again increases to 56% during the third six-month period. During this same time, there is a decrease in numbers of articles requested for these journals through Document Delivery (see Table 3).

Even though there was a 37% decrease in document delivery requests during the study period, overall the library realized a 27% increase in Wiley title usage. During the first six months of the study, Wiley titles were accessed or requested a total of 421 times. During the following year, in that same six-month period, these titles were accessed and requested a total of 536 times.

TABLE 2. Comparison of Web Access Management with Vendor Statistics for Wiley InterScience

	Wiley InterScience				
Month	Off-Campus WAM	Total WAM	% of Off-Campus Use	Vendor-Supplied Total	Estimated Number of Off-Campus Article Accesses*
January 2005	45	4,102	0.01	293	3
February 2005	0	7,054	0	375	0
March 2005	0	7,267	0	385	0
April 2005	330	9,866	0.03	504	15
May 2005	204	7,264	0.03	352	11
June 2005	124	1,772	0.07	302	21
July 2005	274	1,472	0.19	255	48
August 2005	186	1,446	0.13	226	29
September 2005	390	3,928	0.1	270	27
October 2005	815	8,797	0.09	468	42
November 2005	372	16,980	0.02	491	10
December 2005	246	3,876	0.06	265	16
January 2006	3,128	21,560	0.15	389	58
February 2006	2,839	25,685	0.11	475	52
March 2006	1,458	24,356	0.06	461	28
April 2006	1,114	34,074	0.03	605	18
May 2006	3,009	18,031	0.17	467	79
June 2006	3,839	14,885	0.26	259	67
Total	18,373	212,415	0.09	6,842	616

* Rounded to the nearest whole number

TABLE 3. Comparison of Wiley InterScience and Document Delivery in Six-Month Increments

Time Period	Online	Document Delivery	% of Total Accessed Online
Jan.-June 2005	50	371	12%
July-Dec. 2005	172	228	43%
Jan.-June 2006	302	234	56%

Project MUSE

The Project MUSE numbers do not show as clear a trend of increasing or decreasing online usage. The overall percentage of off-campus use during the study period was 3%. This number fluctuated from month to month, peaking at 17% in June 2005 (see Table 4). The July to December 2005 time period in the study revealed the highest online usage, at 180 articles, an increase of 186% from the January to June 2005 time period. During the January to June 2006 time period, online usage decreased by 53%. During the first six months of the study, 39% of off-campus usage was from online access. This increased to 63% during the second six months, and then decreased to 56% in the third six-month period (see Table 5). Comparing the January to June 2005 period to the January to June 2006 time period, there was a 33% increase in online usage and 23% decrease in document delivery requests for the same titles.

DISCUSSION

While this study's numbers only estimate online usage, based on these findings, it appears that off-campus students are beginning to find their own way to full-text material online. While usage of only two online journal packages was examined, it is evident from the decrease in document delivery requests and increase in online access statistics, that more students are satisfying their information needs without the mediated service. Exactly what students are downloading and whether they find the online self-service options user-friendly are still unknowns.

More research needs to be done on how students are interacting with the digital library. There are still a number of requests coming through document delivery for items available online in full text. It would be useful to determine if these students are requesting mediated article delivery because they are having difficulty navigating through the library's online catalog and databases to find full text, are dealing with connectivity or access problems, or if they just prefer the "one-stop" option of ordering everything through one place. These students may be finding citations without ever using the library's databases, through mediated librarian searches or using another university or local public library's resources. If this is the case, it is possible that Central Michigan University students do not realize the wealth of full-text online material available to them. Understanding the reasons behind why students still order these documents could help librarians target their educational and marketing efforts.

Another area for further investigation is whether students and other users feel they sacrifice quality for convenience in the use of online materials. If an article is available online now, is that more important than if the better source would take two days or a week to obtain? This

TABLE 4. Comparison of Web Access Management with Vendor Statistics for Project MUSE

| | Project MUSE | | | | |
Month	Off-Campus WAM	Total WAM	% of Off-Campus Use	Vendor-Supplied Total	Estimated Number of Off-Campus Article Accesses*
January 2005	200	1,329	0.15	139	21
February 2005	20	2,719	0.01	379	4
March 2005	41	2,114	0.02	290	6
April 2005	78	2,912	0.03	428	13
May 2005	4	721	0.01	176	2
June 2005	54	325	0.17	100	17
July 2005	0	769	0	152	0
August 2005	67	570	0.12	121	15
September 2005	22	2,605	0.01	468	5
October 2005	289	3,710	0.08	975	78
November 2005	286	3,947	0.07	956	67
December 2005	52	1,974	0.03	489	15
January 2006	380	5,342	0.07	283	20
February 2006	257	10,811	0.02	664	13
March 2006	345	12,290	0.03	621	19
April 2006	263	16,006	0.02	791	16
May 2006	62	4,881	0.01	306	3
June 2006	233	3,445	0.07	181	13
Total	2,653	76,470	0.03	7,519	226

* Rounded to the nearest whole number

TABLE 5. Comparison of Project MUSE and Document Delivery in Six-Month Increments

Time Period	Online	Document Delivery	% of Total Accessed Online
Jan.-June 2005	63	99	39%
July-Dec. 2005	180	104	63%
Jan.-June 2006	84	76	53%

certainly may depend on the assignment and the amount of time students have to complete it. In Central Michigan University's off-campus settings, students take classes in compressed formats and may not have the luxury of waiting for the best resource if something else more convenient is available now.

This study could be expanded to see whether the trends noted with Wiley and Project MUSE are replicated across all other online journal packages. Noting the use may provide further justification for continued online collection development and a movement to online only journal access.

This study did not investigate whether there was a difference in how on- and off-campus users interact with the digital library. While comparison is difficult in this area as on-campus students do not have access to the mediated document delivery provide by Off-Campus Library Services, it would be interesting to see if one group tends to be more independent than another and what might account for any differences. Also, it would be useful to know if the trend found at Central Michigan University is evident at other institutions. This could help other academic libraries plan for changes in their own specialized services and collection development policies.

CONCLUSION

As shown in this study, identifying ways of accurately counting online usage can be extremely complex. While Central Michigan University Library staff keep a number of electronic statistics, WAM data, Web page access counts, vendor-supplied numbers, etc., there is no clear best practice for determining one use of a resource. Each source counts in a different way. As the trend continues toward a more robust electronic collection, there is a definite need to develop better methods of tracking use in order to make informed collection development decisions.

OpenURL linking products such as Ex Libris™ SFX® or Serials Solutions Article Linker™ may also contribute to standardized internal tracking in the future. Central Michigan University Library began implementation of an OpenURL linker early in 2006. It is expected that the data generated from this linker will provide a more consistent and reliable picture of online use. Since implementation was very recent, there is not sufficient data to begin analyzing the usefulness of the information captured through this product.

Another option to explore is writing filters for the WAM proxy server. The filters are specifically programmed elements that look for matching sequences in the hypertext source code for each and every resource to be tracked. Setting up filters is complicated and time-consuming. The source code for each resource has to be analyzed and the corresponding filter specifically written so that the data is collected and counted in the same way. This alternative requires careful study to determine if the data would be unique and valuable enough to justify the efforts needed to create it. No matter what the solution, it will make comparison with past data difficult, posing yet additional questions about how the library analyzes trends for collection development and management.

REFERENCES

1. Calvert, H.M. "The Impact of Electronic Journals and Aggregate Databases on Interlibrary Loan: A Case Study at Ball State University Libraries." *New Library World* 101, no. 1153 (2000): 28-31.

2. Solar, D. "Electronic Full-Text Articles as a Substitute for Traditional Interlibrary Borrowing." *Journal of Interlibrary Loan, Document Delivery, and Information Supply* 11, no. 1 (2000): 99-118.

3. Kidd, T. "Does Electronic Journal Access Affect Document Delivery Requests? Some Data from Glasgow University Library." *Interlending and Document Supply* 31, no. 4 (2003): 264-9.

4. Yue, P.W., and Syring, M.L. "Usage of Electronic Journals and Their Effect on Interlibrary Loan: A Case Study at the University of Nevada, Reno." *Library Collections, Acquisitions, and Technical Services* 28(2004): 420-32.

5. Echeverria, M., and Barredo, P. "Online Journals: Their Impact on Document Delivery." *Interlending and Document Supply* 33, no. 3 (2005): 145-9.

6. Egan, N. "The Impact of Electronic Full-Text Resources on Interlibrary Loan: A Ten Year Study at John Jay College of Criminal Justice." *Journal of Interlibrary Loan, Document Delivery, and Electronic Reserve* 15, no. 3 (2005): 23-41.

doi:10.1300/J383v04n01_08

Integrating E-Resources into an Online Catalog: The Hospital Library Experience

Devica Ramjit Samsundar

SUMMARY. In today's Internet-friendly world, an online catalog is considered a "standard" resource in most libraries. Some medical librarians have a difficult time meeting that expectation, as their libraries tend to be understaffed and ill-equipped to tackle a project of such magnitude. This article gives a detailed account of how librarians at Baptist Health South Florida migrated from a traditional catalog to a robust, interactive, Web-based online catalog. This account focuses on their experience selecting software, creating an infrastructure, collecting and organizing e-resources, communicating with vendors, and understanding MARC tag 856. doi:10.1300/ J383v04n01_09 *[Article copies available for a fee from The Haworth Document Delivery Service: 1-800-HAWORTH. E-mail address: <docdelivery@haworthpress.com> Website: <http://www.HaworthPress.com> © 2007 by The Haworth Press, Inc. All rights reserved.]*

KEYWORDS. OPAC, hospital libraries, cataloging, electronic resources, TAG 856

Devica Ramjit Samsundar, MLIS (devicas@baptisthealth.net) is Electronic Services Librarian at Baptist Health South Florida, South Miami Hospital, 6200 SW 73 Street, Miami, FL 33143.

[Haworth co-indexing entry note]: "Integrating E-Resources into an Online Catalog: The Hospital Library Experience." Samsundar, Devica Ramjit. Co-published simultaneously in the *Journal of Electronic Resources in Medical Libraries* (The Haworth Information Press, an imprint of The Haworth Press, Inc.) Vol. 4, No. 1/2, 2007, pp. 87-99; and: *Electronic Resources in Medical Libraries: Issues and Solutions* (ed: Elizabeth Connor, and M. Sandra Wood) The Haworth Information Press, an imprint of The Haworth Press, Inc., 2007, pp. 87-99. Single or multiple copies of this article are available for a fee from The Haworth Document Delivery Service [1-800-HAWORTH, 9:00 a.m. - 5:00 p.m. (EST). E-mail address: docdelivery@haworthpress.com].

Available online at http://jerml.haworthpress.com
© 2007 by The Haworth Press, Inc. All rights reserved.
doi:10.1300/J383v04n01_09

INTRODUCTION

With the advances that the Internet has brought to many aspects of daily life, the mindset of many people is "technology equals instant gratification." They expect banks to allow online transactions, gas stations to allow pay at the pump, and all retail stores to have an online equivalent. These expectations do not stop at the library doors. Users want e-books, e-journals, and databases to easily locate the information that they want 24/7. Within the hospital library sector, patron needs are not only driven by the change in culture, but by health care practitioners who need information at their fingertips for the delivery of quality patient care.

At Baptist Health South Florida, the librarians recognized the need for e-content and responded to clientele wishes. In 1997, the electronic medical library made its debut on the hospital's intranet by highlighting the small collection of e-journals and e-books from Ovid Technologies, under the heading "Electronic Medical Library." In the years that followed, librarians utilized usage statistics and patron feedback in order to continuously develop this e-collection. Today, resources from aggregators such as MD Consult, EBSCO Health Business, and PubMed Central have been integrated into the library's intranet. The entire library section of the intranet is now referred to as the "Electronic Medical Library."

OPAC or Not to OPAC

As the collection of e-books and e-journals grew, it became increasingly difficult for the staff to memorize the collection and to know which vendor, aggregator, or source contained the item that was needed. Needless to say, this was also a problem for library patrons. It became apparent that there was a need to merge all e-content into one resource. The librarians realized that implementing an Online Public Access Catalog (OPAC) was the logical solution for the following reasons:

- Staff and patrons would have access to the catalog from their PC desktop so there would be no more guessing which materials the library owned.
- Hyperlinks could be embedded in the catalog to allow users to link directly to the source.
- Catalog records for print materials in the library collection would promote use of the physical library.
- The entire collection would be searchable by subject, author, or title.

Despite the obvious advantages of having an online catalog, librarians were still reluctant to take on such an ambitious project. At the time, the library staff consisted of a library director, electronic resources librarian, one full-time senior library technician, and three part-time library support staff. The six staff members were responsible for delivering library services to 10,000 hospital employees and 2,000 physicians affiliated with Baptist Health South Florida. The librarians thought adding one more project seemed overwhelming and unrealistic. Additionally, both librarians had limited experience dealing with original cataloging and were not accustomed to working with MARC records. In the past, only a small number of books required original cataloging. Most catalog cards were purchased from MARCIVE for about a dollar a record. With affordable catalog cards and being relatively understaffed, librarians also questioned the return on investment. The preconceived notion was it would take months to convert the paper records into MARC records, and it would be a horrendous task to code the e-resources into the catalog, leading to the question of whether the library really needed an OPAC.

The librarians also considered implementing an A-Z e-resources list. The listing would satisfy the need to consolidate the entire collection and allow users to link to online resources. However, it would be a static page and would not allow users to do any type of dynamic searching. Although an A-Z list would be a less demanding solution, the librarians realized it was not a viable option, considering the exponential growth of their e-resources.

OPAC, Now What?

After careful consideration of the pros and cons, the librarians decided to strive for excellence and automate the card catalog. The library director did the initial research on the various software vendors by consulting with colleges, reviewing the literature, and test-driving online catalogs that were powered by the various serials management systems. Vendors were evaluated based on the technical specifications shown in Figure 1. The key components were: Application Service Provider (ASP) Web hosting, ability to handle multiple collections, and the capability to link to e-journals and e-books.

With ASP Web hosting, the responsibility for data security, file storage, and hardware/software updates resides with the vendor, thereby minimizing the need for assistance from the hospital's information technology (IT) department. IT's typical concerns related to network

FIGURE 1. Software Specification Checklist

❑ASP Web hosting
❑Integrates MARCIVE records
❑Capable of handling multiple library locations
❑Links to e-journals
❑OpenURL for link resolution from databases
   such as Ovid, EBSCOhost, and MD Consult
❑Check-in journals
❑Claims Management - with warnings for missing
   issues.
❑Displays serials holdings
❑Customized OPAC interfaces
❑Ability to search via MeSH subject headings,
   keyword, author, title, subject heading, call
   number. Search results can be displayed,
   e-mailed, or printed.
❑URL tester from OPAC
❑Ability to run reports (claims)

security, financial obligations, and ongoing data maintenance would be diminished. Their main involvement in the migration process would be to authorize IP authentication to the catalog from all PCs on the Baptist Health South Florida network.

The capability of accommodating collections from multiple locations was a crucial component that could not to be compromised. Baptist Health South Florida has three libraries that are accessible to all Baptist Health employees: Marmot Foundation Health Sciences located at South Miami Hospital, Jaffee Medical Library at the Baptist Hospital campus, and the virtual library on the intranet. There is some overlap in the book and journal collections at each library; nonetheless, collections vary based on the needs of their constituents. Having software that allows users to know the availability of an item and their options for access would promote usage across the health system. For instance, the Jaffee Library houses the majority of the pediatric collection because it is on the same campus as the Baptist Children's Hospital. Although the materials reside at that library, they can be checked out and sent by interoffice mail to an employee at another campus. Furthermore, if a resource were available electronically, the patron should be able to link directly to it regardless of physical location.

After months of research, the librarians chose CyberTools for Libraries as their integrated library system and OPAC vendor. CyberTools satisfied all of their technical specifications plus offered a robust search engine that allowed for MeSH searching. Additionally, the company has considerable experience working with medical libraries and was highly recommended by the library director at Orlando Regional Hospital.

Knowing the magnitude of the task at hand, the project was shared between the two librarians. Diane Rourke, library service director, was responsible for converting the physical book and journal collection. Devica Samsundar, electronic resources librarian, was in charge of integrating the electronic titles into the OPAC. Both librarians enlisted the assistance of support staff. By involving the library technicians at the ground level, the librarians were certain to gain support once the system was in place.

CONVERTING THE PHYSICAL COLLECTION

Moving from a card catalog and manual journal check-in to a Web-based OPAC required a lot of dedication. The project began with the library director leading the transformation of the physical book and journal collection that she developed over the previous 30 years. She worked closely with the technical support departments at CyberTools and MARCIVE to explore all the conversion options, assessing each for efficiency and cost effectiveness. For a small fee, MARCIVE provided the records for the 3,000 books that were purchased over the last three decades. Librarians and library staff pored through the records to delete the ones that were no longer in the collection. Once the editing was completed, MARCIVE transferred the remaining records into the catalog, and the MARC records were manually edited to reflect location (campus, reference, circulation, etc.) information.

To integrate the library's 300 print journal subscriptions, CyberTools uploaded the institution's SERHOLD records into the catalog. Ms. Rourke then manipulated the records to reflect the expected received date, journal frequency, and volume/issue number. Once that information was programmed into CyberTools, the check-in and claiming process became totally computerized. Staff no longer had to manually review the check-in cards for missing issues, and from any PC within Baptist Health the staff could view if the latest issue of their favorite journal had been received in the library.

Integrating the Electronic Collection

With the physical collection in the catalog, it was the electronic re-sources librarian's turn to venture into the cataloging world by design-ing and implementing a systematic way to integrate the e-collection into the OPAC. The success of this portion depended on the "planning stage." Many hours were dedicated to selecting the infrastructure and gathering/collecting all e-resources. Additionally, she needed to fully understand the 856 tag and its capabilities in order to import more than 900 e-journals and more than 100 e-books.

Separate Records versus Single Record

In cataloging terms, a solid infrastructure started with deciding single versus separate records for e-resources. Single record meant there would be one record for each item in the library, and if the library held the item's electronic equivalent, the 856 tag would be edited to embed the link in its electronic record. With separate records, there would be two records in the catalog for print and electronic versions of an item. One would give all the pertinent information (call number, availability, etc.) for the physical book. The second, would link to the electronic text.

To further clarify the single record approach, if a library owned both an electronic and print copy of *Harrison's Principles of Internal Medicine,* users searching the catalog would see only one record for *Harrison's* as shown in Figure 2. Within that record they would see that an electronic edition was available. Clicking on the embedded URL would connect them to the electronic version of the book.

Knowing the ramifications of this decision between single and sepa-rate records, the electronic resources librarian did a comprehensive search for existing guidelines. The guidelines/recommendations from Cooper-ative Online Serials (CONSER) and OCLC were consulted.

CONSER Working Group recommends a single record for any of the following situations:

- Equivalent content: the content of the paper and electronic versions are the same but the titles differ.

FIGURE 2. OPAC Record for *Harrison's Principles of Internal Medicine*

```
Medical Library
Details: 1 of 1. 30 lines.

   Search Results  |  Main  | Help |
──────────────────────────────────────────────────────────────────────────

WB      Harrison's principles of internal medicine.  -- 16th ed. / editors, Dennis
115     L. Kasper ... [et al.]  -- New York : McGraw-Hill, Medical Pub. Division,
H322    c2005.
2005    xxvii, [2750] p. : ill. (some col.), col. maps ; 29 cm.
           Includes bibliographical references and index.
           Introduction to clinical medicine -- Cardinal manifestations and
        presentation of diseases -- Genetics and disease -- Nutrition -- Oncology
        and hematology -- Infectious diseases -- Bioterrorism and clinical
        medicine -- Disorders of the cardiovascular system -- Disorders of the
        respiratory system -- Critical care medicine -- Disorders of the kidney
        and urinary tract -- Disorders of the gastrointestinal system -- Disorders
        of the immune system, connective tissue, and joints -- Endocrinology and
        metabolism -- Neurologic disorders -- Poisoning, drug overdose, and
        envenomation.
           1. Internal medicine.  2. Internal Medicine.  I. Kasper, Dennis L.
        II. Harrison, Tinsley Randolph, 1900- Principles of internal medicine.
        III. Principles of internal medicine.

        This item is also available electronically!  Online access restricted to
        Baptist Health South Florida IP address; User ID and Password required off
        campus.
        Link to online text.

Volume/Issue/Year/Copy       Location  Call#              Status
V=1/C=1                      SM REF                        available
V=2/C=1                      SM REF                        available
V=1/C=2                      BH REF                        available
V=2                          BH REF                        available
```

- Equivalent content with different presentation (e.g., articles are added to an issue by the publisher as soon as they are ready, rather than releasing complete issue).
- Titles of the print and electronic versions change simultaneously.
- Government Printing Office (GPO) single-record copy is available.[3]

CONSER Working Group recommends separate records for any of the following situations:

- Resource exists only in electronic form.
- Content of electronic resource differs significantly from print resource.
- Resource undergoes a change in format, usually from print to electronic.
- Resource is a database or Web site whose content is equivalent to more than one print source (e.g., Web of Science).
- Resource is a database or Web site whose content includes significant new material beyond existing print sources.
- Original text cannot be definitively identified.[3]

OCLC states that creating separate records for an item is preferable when both remote access electronic versions and tangible or direct access (including, but not limited to, print and other non-electronic) versions exist. However, they recommend verifying the impact of single versus double record with your local system vendor and other partners prior to deciding on a format.[7]

After the research was concluded, it was decided to use the single record option and add the MARC 856 tag to link to online resources. This option was advantageous to Baptist Health because the e-books and e-journals that were in question were all equivalent in content to their hard copy counterpart. With this choice, users would be able to view all access points from one record, therefore eliminating the need to go back and forth between records. For example, if the patron checks the availability of the most recent issue of *New England Journal of Medicine*, as shown in Figure 3, he or she can see which issues are available in the library and at the same time, click to connect to the online journal.

MARC Tags

When cataloging, it is important to put the entire project into perspective. The librarian controls what the patrons will ultimately see and use

FIGURE 3. *New England Journal of Medicine*–Single Record View

```
Medical Library
Details: 1 of 1. 24 lines.

  Main |  Help |


SHELVED    The New England journal of medicine. Massachusetts Medical Society.
WITH           -- v. 198-        Feb. 23, 1928-     .  -- Boston, Massachusetts
JOURNALS   Medical Society.
             v. illus., ports.
             Weekly
             Also available online. Password required for access.
             Continues the Boston medical and surgical journal.
             1. Medicine--Periodicals  2. Online journal

             This item is also available electronically!  Online access restricted
             to Baptist Health South Florida IP address; User ID and Password
             required off campus.
             Link to online text.

Latest issue received on 05/24/06:
  Yr: 2006  Vol: 354  Iss: 21  Mon: MAY  Day: 25
Copy 1:
  Hold: SM 1998- : 338-
  HOLD: 2005-2006 : 352N1-12,14-26/353/354N1-21/
Copy 2:
  Hold: BH 2003 : 348-
  HOLD: 2005-2006 : 352N1-13,15-16,18-26/353N1-17,19-26/354N1-21/


  Browse Holdings  |  Volumes |
```

through the 856 field. MARC21 field 856 is used to specify location and access information for an electronic resource.[6] To create the cross-linking as shown in Figures 2 and 3, librarians edited the 856 tag and subfield $u, $y and $z. Figure 4 shows the CyberTools back-office view, where fields can be edited. Subfield $u represents the real resource URL provided by the vendor. Subfield $y houses the text that masks the URL and $z is the public note to users.[5]

Additionally, MARC tag 099 (the local call number field) was edited when items were available solely in the electronic collection (see Figure 5). Keying "online journal" or "online book" into subfield $a, within MARC tag 099, allows users to clearly distinguish the online-only text, or query the catalog for full-text content.

Gathering and Organizing E-Resources

Once the infrastructure was set up, the next step was to organize all of the e-books and e-journals. At that point, the library had institutional

FIGURE 4. CyberTool User Screen for 856 Tag

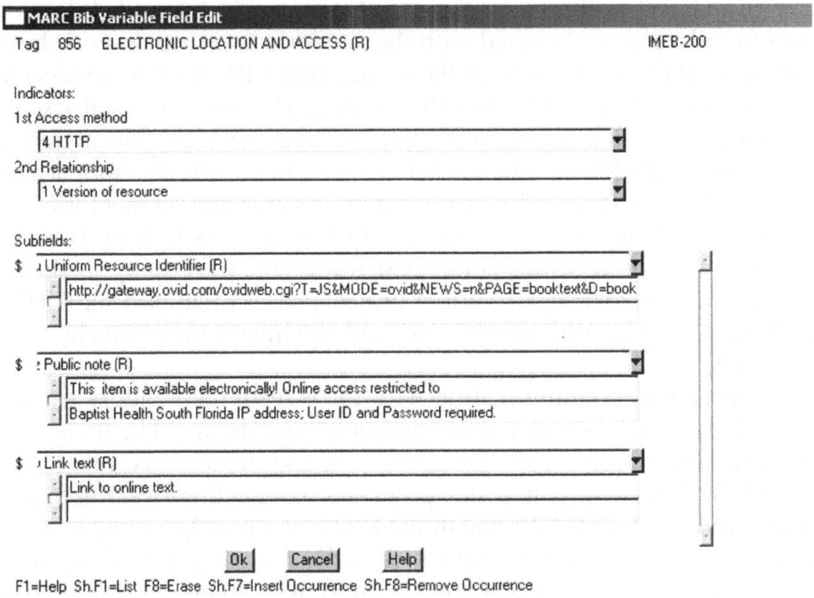

FIGURE 5. OPAC View When 099 Tag Is Edited

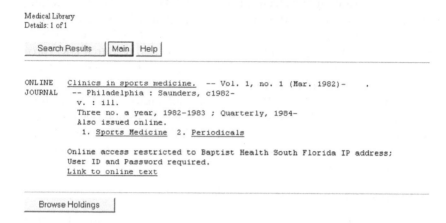

subscriptions to over 900 electronic titles from Ovid, MD Consult, and EBSCO Health Business Elite. To consolidate the titles, the librarian created an Excel workbook, as shown in Figure 6, which included all titles held for all vendors. Labeled with the vendor's name, each worksheet captured details such as title of the item, direct URL, and the necessary steps to integrate the item into the catalog. The librarian used Excel, rather than Access, to track/collect the information because the majority of vendors send URL information in Excel or comma delimited format, eliminating the need to recreate/transfer the information into another format.

The worksheet was also used as a communication tool. As portions of the integration project were completed, it was noted. By doing so, the librarian was able to delegate various project phases to support staff. This in turn prevented duplication of work and maximized the efforts by support staff.

Furthermore, communicating with the e-resource vendors and/or publishers saved a tremendous amount of man-hours. The technical support departments were all eager to help and in most cases they had already facilitated the conversion processes of other libraries. Important information such as ISBNs and direct URLs was readily available. Furnishing this information to libraries was also beneficial for the vendor, because once the item was embedded into the catalog, the OPAC became another portal to their materials.

FIGURE 6. Excel Workbook Used to Organize All E-Resources

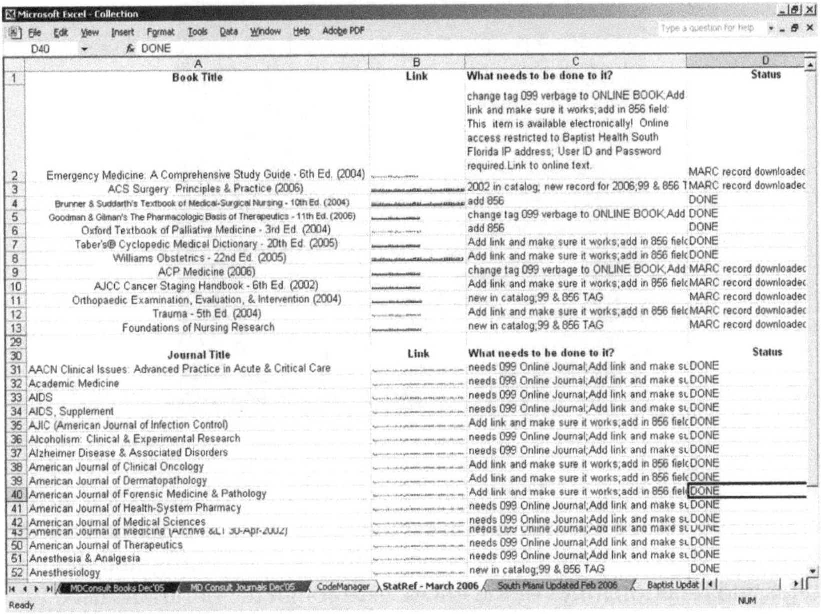

Microsoft Excel - Collection

D40 DONE

	A	B	C	D
1	**Book Title**	**Link**	**What needs to be done to it?**	**Status**
2	Emergency Medicine: A Comprehensive Study Guide - 6th Ed. (2004)		change tag 099 verbage to ONLINE BOOK;Add link and make sure it works;add in 856 field: This item is available electronically! Online access restricted to Baptist Health South Florida IP address; User ID and Password required.Link to online text.	MARC record downloadec
3	ACS Surgery: Principles & Practice (2006)		2002 in catalog; new record for 2006;99 & 856 T	MARC record downloadec
4	Brunner & Suddarth's Textbook of Medical-Surgical Nursing - 10th Ed. (2004)		add 856	DONE
5	Goodman & Gilman's The Pharmacologic Basis of Therapeutics - 11th Ed. (2006)		change tag 099 verbage to ONLINE BOOK;Add	DONE
6	Oxford Textbook of Palliative Medicine - 3rd Ed. (2004)		add 856	DONE
7	Taber's® Cyclopedic Medical Dictionary - 20th Ed. (2005)		Add link and make sure it works;add in 856 fielc	DONE
8	Williams Obstetrics - 22nd Ed. (2005)		Add link and make sure it works;add in 856 fielc	DONE
9	ACP Medicine (2006)		change tag 099 verbage to ONLINE BOOK;Add	MARC record downloadec
10	AJCC Cancer Staging Handbook - 6th Ed. (2002)		Add link and make sure it works;add in 856 fielc	MARC record downloadec
11	Orthopaedic Examination, Evaluation, & Intervention (2004)		new in catalog;99 & 856 TAG	MARC record downloadec
12	Trauma - 5th Ed. (2004)		Add link and make sure it works;add in 856 fielc	MARC record downloadec
13	Foundations of Nursing Research		new in catalog;99 & 856 TAG	MARC record downloadec
29				
30	**Journal Title**	**Link**	**What needs to be done to it?**	**Status**
31	AACN Clinical Issues: Advanced Practice in Acute & Critical Care		needs 099 Online Journal;Add link and make su	DONE
32	Academic Medicine		needs 099 Online Journal;Add link and make su	DONE
33	AIDS		needs 099 Online Journal;Add link and make su	DONE
34	AIDS, Supplement		needs 099 Online Journal;Add link and make su	DONE
35	AJIC (American Journal of Infection Control)		Add link and make sure it works;add in 856 fielc	DONE
36	Alcoholism: Clinical & Experimental Research		needs 099 Online Journal;Add link and make su	DONE
37	Alzheimer Disease & Associated Disorders		needs 099 Online Journal;Add link and make su	DONE
38	American Journal of Clinical Oncology		Add link and make sure it works;add in 856 fielc	DONE
39	American Journal of Dermatopathology		Add link and make sure it works;add in 856 fielc	DONE
40	American Journal of Forensic Medicine & Pathology		Add link and make sure it works;add in 856 fiel	DONE
41	American Journal of Health-System Pharmacy		needs 099 Online Journal;Add link and make su	DONE
42	American Journal of Medical Sciences		needs 099 Online Journal;Add link and make su	DONE
43	American Journal of Medicine (Archive &LT 30-Apr-2002)		needs 099 Online Journal;Add link and make su	DONE
50	American Journal of Therapeutics		needs 099 Online Journal;Add link and make su	DONE
51	Anesthesia & Analgesia		needs 099 Online Journal;Add link and make su	DONE
52	Anesthesiology		new in catalog;99 & 856 TAG	DONE

MDConsult Books Dec'05 / MD Consult Journals Dec'05 / CodeManager / StatRef - March 2006 / South Miami Updated Feb 2006 / Baptist Updat

Ready NUM

With the help of the staff and working closely with the vendors, librarians integrated the e-resources into the catalog in roughly three months. If the staff had been able to dedicate their full attention to the cataloging project, it could have been finished in fewer than two months. Nevertheless, cataloging is a detail-oriented set of tasks that requires intense and prolonged focus on the PC that can become monotonous. It is best to set realistic goals and pace the work. By doing so, the staff can stay focused and keep errors to a minimum.

Promote the Catalog

Once the initial migration was completed, the librarians used the intranet to promote the catalog's availability. In order to make a lasting impression, the library director converted an old catalog drawer into a planter box as shown in Figure 7. She then used it as a prop during presentations to highlight that the library had moved away from the old card catalog system. The library staff made the old cards available to

FIGURE 7. Catalog Drawer Planter

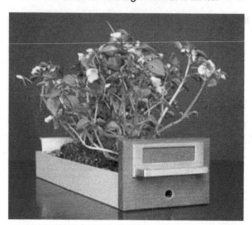

patrons as scrap paper. The electronic resources librarian took a different approach. She created a PowerPoint presentation patterned on the Extreme Makeover television program theme that highlighted the features and functionalities of the OPAC. Although the librarians used two drastically different approaches, they had a unified goal of bringing visibility to the catalog.

CONCLUSION

Conversion of the card catalog and the integration of the e-collection into the catalog was just the beginning. The OPAC has the potential of becoming a "one-stop source" at Baptist Health for e-books and e-journals. Several departments have purchased institutional subscriptions to resources such as online dictionaries, JCAHO publications, and e-books, all of which permit direct linking. By adding those titles to the catalog, the OPAC serves as an e-resource repository that masks details such as vendor information and URLs behind the facade of the card catalog. Additionally, as a result of making the resource readily available to the entire organization, the OPAC maximizes the institution's return on investment.

Health care practitioners need to access reliable information on a 24/7 basis in order to continuously deliver quality care. Medical librarians can satisfy that need by migrating from a card catalog to an interactive online catalog that links to e-books and e-journals. If the transition does not occur, users will view the library as an inadequate "thing of the past" and may turn to "Googling it" for a quick answer. Following the lead of the librarians at Baptist Health South Florida, migrating to an online catalog is an attainable goal. As shown by the Baptist Health experience, the keys to success were researching, planning, and staying focused.

REFERENCES

1. Bothman, R. "Cataloging Electronic Books." *Library Resources & Technical Services* 48, no. 1 (2004): 12-9.

2. Burrows, S. "A Review of Electronic Journal Acquisition, Management, and Use in Health Sciences Libraries." *Journal of the Medical Library Association* 94, no. 1 (2006): 67-74.

3. CONSER Working Group. "Single or Separate Records? What's Appropriate and When." Available: <http://wwwtest.library.ucla.edu/libraries/cataloging/sercat/conserwg>. Accessed: May 15, 2006.

4. Davis, E., and Stone, J. "From A to Z: Automated Catalogue to Web OPAC and Z39.50." *Health Libraries Review* 15, no. 2 (1998):128-32.

5. Fritz, D.A. *Cataloging with AARC2 and MARC21: For Books, Electronic Resources, Sound Recordings, Videorecordings, and Serials*. Chicago, IL: American Library Association, 2004.

6. Library of Congress Network Development and MARC Standards Office. "MARC 21 Formats: Guidelines for the Use of Field 856." Available: <http://www.loc.gov/marc/856guide.html>. Accessed: May 10, 2006.

7. Weitz, J. "Cataloging Electronic Resources: OCLC-MARC Coding Guidelines." Available: <http://www.oclc.org/support/documentation/worldcat/cataloging/electronicresources/>. Accessed: May 15, 2006.

doi:10.1300/ J383v04n01_09

Is There a Pending Change
in Medical Publisher and Library Liability?

A. Bruce Strauch
Earl Walker
Mark Bebensee

SUMMARY. This article addresses the peculiar reluctance of courts to permit suits in negligence and strict liability against publishers for erroneous information that leads to harm. A narrow exception made for airplane landing charts combined with the change in delivery method of medical information is a wedge into medical publishing that will soon eliminate the safe harbor. As medical library Web sites actively participate in electronic delivery, they have the potential to be drawn in as endorsers or actual publishers of erroneous data. doi:10.1300/J383v04n01_10 *[Article copies available for a fee from The Haworth Document Delivery Service: 1-800-HAWORTH. E-mail address: <docdelivery@haworthpress.com> Website: <http://www.HaworthPress.com> © 2007 by The Haworth Press, Inc. All rights reserved.]*

A. Bruce Strauch, MA, JD (strauchb@citadel.edu) is Associate Professor of Business Law, and owner of the scholarly publishing journal *Against the Grain* and The Charleston Information Group, LLC; Earl Walker, PhD (earl.walker@citadel.edu) is Dean and Robert A. Jolly Chair of Leadership and Management; and Mark Bebensee, PhD (mark.bebensee@citadel.edu) is Associate Dean and Associate Professor; all at the School of Business Administration, The Citadel, 171 Moultrie Street, Charleston, SC 29409.

[Haworth co-indexing entry note]: "Is There a Pending Change in Medical Publisher and Library Liability?" Strauch, A. Bruce, Earl Walker, and Mark Bebensee. Co-published simultaneously in the *Journal of Electronic Resources in Medical Libraries* (The Haworth Information Press, an imprint of The Haworth Press, Inc.) Vol. 4, No. 1/2, 2007, pp. 101-112; and: *Electronic Resources in Medical Libraries: Issues and Solutions* (ed: Elizabeth Connor, and M. Sandra Wood) The Haworth Information Press, an imprint of The Haworth Press, Inc., 2007, pp. 101-112. Single or multiple copies of this article are available for a fee from The Haworth Document Delivery Service [1-800-HAWORTH, 9:00 a.m. - 5:00 p.m. (EST). E-mail address: docdelivery@haworthpress.com].

Available online at http://jerml.haworthpress.com
© 2007 by The Haworth Press, Inc. All rights reserved.
doi:10.1300/J383v04n01_10

KEYWORDS. Negligence, products liability, publisher liability, strict tort liability

INTRODUCTION

Aside from defamation, the publishing industry has been virtually immune from suits for erroneous information that leads to injury. While an author may be sued by a victim, case law almost universally leaves the publisher free from liability. The justifications for this range from a defense of free expression, to a fear of burdening the industry with a duty to test products or replicate scientific studies. Scientific and medical publishers do not tend to defame people. Thus, these publishers have enjoyed low insurance costs and presumably broadened profit margins, a state of affairs that may not last for long, given the changing nature of the delivery of published information. The two legal theories that would hold any other industry liable for injury are negligence and strict tort liability.

NEGLIGENCE

Presented as a linear diagram the elements of negligence law are:

(a) Duty (b) Act of Negligence (c) Proximate cause (d) Injury

Generally, one has a duty not to injure people. That duty is quite broad and is activated by any action with foreseeable bad consequences. Next, the nature of the action is examined. Was reasonable care used? Did one act as a reasonably prudent person?[1] Then, did the act of negligence directly or proximately cause the injury? If all elements are present, then one is liable for the injuries.

Under negligence law, whenever one acts, he or she has a duty to look down the road and think about possible dire consequences and modify actions accordingly. Otherwise liability for damages is imposed.[2] The applicability of negligence law to publishing seems as logical as it would to driving an automobile. Yet courts have shut down negligence suits against publishers almost universally with the first element, saying that absent unusual circumstances, publishers have no negligence duty to their readers. If the publisher has no duty to the reader, then the chain of elements does not begin. It simply doesn't matter if a publisher can foresee injury to a reader if the information is flawed.

Birmingham vs. Fodor's Travel Publications, Inc.[3] is an emblematic case. The book in question was Fodor's *Hawaii 1988*, which provided a guide to the Hawaiian Islands. A honeymooning couple claimed to have used the guide to direct them to a beach where the husband was hit by savage waves while swimming and sustained injuries. The Supreme Court of Hawaii dismissed the lawsuit with the first element of negligence, holding no publication owed a duty to a reader unless the publisher authored or guaranteed the information.[4]

Is Editing Authoring?

In *Jones vs. J.B. Lippincott Co.,*[5] a nursing student was injured after treating herself for constipation with a hydrogen peroxide enema. Her source for this curative was the *Textbook for Medical and Surgical Nursing,* 5th edition, published by J. B. Lippincott Company. The court held that publishing the work of one of its own employees would hold the publisher liable under agency law of *respondeat superior.* Otherwise the publisher has no duty as to the book's contents.[6] The logic of agency law is that a company has control over employees and should be liable for injuries they cause.

Interestingly, the plaintiff argued that the work of a Lippincott editor made the publisher a co-author. To the contrary, the editor did the usual tasks of reading for clarity and organization and making suggestions that frequently were not followed. In other words, she edited and did not author the work.[7]

When Does a Publisher Guarantee?

In *Walters vs. Seventeen Magazine,*[8] a teenager suffered toxic shock after using a Playtex tampon advertised in this popular magazine. The California Court of Appeals found that the magazine did not endorse the advertised product and made no promotional effort beyond running the advertising. Without an endorsement designed to induce a purchase, there is no liability.[9]

In a creative bit of lawyering, the plaintiff's attorney argued that *Seventeen's* actions amounted to an endorsement. It positioned the ad among articles on puberty, gynecology, and menstruation, thereby confusing the immature teenage mind with the mix of fact and hype. The court dismissed this claim, saying that "a small child" could distinguish one from the other.[10] Not addressed in the holding was what result a true confusion or blurring of fact with hype might bring.

More importantly, the court distinguished the facts from *Hanberry vs. Hearst Corp.*,[11] where the plaintiff bought a pair of "slip-proof" shoes bearing the famous "*Good Housekeeping's* Consumer Guaranty Seal," slipped, fell, and was injured. If the guaranty language was not enough, the seal read: "We satisfy ourselves that products advertised in *Good Housekeeping* are good ones and that the advertising claims made for them in our magazine are truthful."[12]

The court held *Good Housekeeping* endorsed the product for its own economic gain, encouraging the consumer to buy both the product and the magazine to learn of other guaranteed products. It "in effect loaned its reputation to promote and induce the sale of a given product..."[13] This imposed a duty of reasonable care.

The *Walters vs. Seventeen* court clearly stated the public policy of no duty absent an endorsement. Advertising liability of the proposed nature, it said, would require magazines to maintain huge testing staffs for each product. This exorbitant cost would drastically raise the cost of ads, killing advertising and ultimately magazines themselves.[14]

PRODUCTS LIABILITY–STRICT TORT

The industrial revolution brought a vast array of manufactured products onto the market, some of which caused injuries without redress under a theory of negligence. The bankrupt manufacturer or else one who went beyond reasonable care and had state-of-the-art equipment are holes in negligence liability. In the first case, there is no one to sue; in the second, the manufacturer has not been negligent.

What economists call a "spill-over cost" was imposed on society via the injured consumer. If the consumer lacked insurance, then society had to pick up the tab through social welfare or government regulation. To correct this lack of protection, strict tort, or products liability as it is popularly called, was developed.[15]

The objective of strict tort was to put the cost back on the manufacturer by forcing him to buy products liability insurance; this premium was then paid by the consumer at purchase through some small part of the price.[16] The model was Section 402A of the *Restatement (Second) of Torts.*[17] Manufacturers were to be "strictly liable," which is to say liable without a showing of negligence. Eliminated were both the state-of-the-art defense and the difficulty of finding the act of negligence in a tangled stream of commerce.

The diagram of elements now became:

(a) Duty (b) Defect   (c) Unreasonable (d) Proximate (e) Injury
                       Danger   Cause

     1. design   ambush
     2. manufacturing
     3. failure to warn

To deal with the bankrupt manufacturer problem, all sellers in the stream of commerce were made liable. This forced manufacturer, wholesaler, and retailer to purchase products liability insurance.

The focus was now on a defect in the product. Defects were classified as either a design or manufacturing defect, or a failure to warn. While many products are defective, the defect in question had to make the product unreasonably dangerous. This is to say that the consumer was ambushed by something he did not reasonably expect, hence the importance of warnings and the current plethora of often elementary warnings on products.

In 1963, California led the way in adopting products liability in *Greenman vs. Yuba Power Products, Inc.*[18] Some variety of Section 402A has subsequently been adopted in statutory form by legislatures or recognized by the appellate courts in nearly all states.[19]

Information Not a Product

Confronted with the strict tort theory of liability, courts have universally declared that information is not a product. *Smith vs. Linn*[20] involved a liquid protein diet promoted by a book entitled, *When Everything Else Fails ... The Last Chance Diet.* Following a woman's death from cardiac failure, her estate sued the publisher Lyle Stuart, Inc. for products liability. Plaintiff asserted the diet book was a defective product such as was contemplated by the products liability statute of the state. The court flatly rejected this, saying that no appellate court in any jurisdiction has held a book to be a product of that nature, and at that time, two courts had expressly stated it was not.[21] Of the two cases cited, most notable was *Cardozo vs. True*,[22] which distinguished between the binding and pages of a book, which is a product, and the ideas, which are not.

Cardozo involved the book *Tradewinds Cookery*, which failed to warn that uncooked Dasheen plants were poisonous, thereby causing a reader to suffer agonizing stomach cramps. The court was particularly bothered by the liability of all firms in the stream of commerce that strict tort imposes:

> It is unthinkable that standards imposed on the quality of goods sold by a merchant would require that merchant, who is a book seller, to evaluate the thought processes of the many authors and publishers of the hundreds and often thousands of books which the merchant offers for sale. One can readily imagine the extent of potential litigation. Is the newsdealer, or for that matter the neighborhood news carrier, liable if the local paper's recipes call for inedible ingredients? We think not.[23]

Winter vs. G.P. Putnam's Sons[24] has a truly horrifying set of facts. *The Encyclopedia of Mushrooms* is a reference guide on picking and cooking wild mushrooms. Plaintiffs relied on the book, ate something deadly poisonous, and suffered critical illness requiring liver transplants. The Ninth Circuit insisted that products liability applied only to tangible items such as automobile tires and not the "unique characteristics of ideas and expression."[25] In examining the public policy behind it all, the court was particularly disturbed by a potential chilling effect on the exchange of ideas. It noted that innovation of new products might be inhibited by strict tort, but found this far "less disturbing than the prospect that we might be deprived of the latest ideas and theories,"[25] and went on to state:

> We place a high priority on the unfettered exchange of ideas. We accept the risk that words and ideas have wings we cannot clip and which carry them we know not where. The threat of liability without fault (financial responsibility for our words and ideas in the absence of fault or a special undertaking or responsibility) could seriously inhibit those who wish to share thoughts and theories.[25]

Free Expression Gets Thrown In

The Ninth Circuit is not alone in its fear of stifling the free flow of ideas should strict tort be applied to publishers and information sellers. Most cases also weave in free speech concerns. Citing a fear of chilling free expression and speech, the *Jones vs. Lippincott* court held strict liability inapplicable to "an idea or knowledge in books or other published material."[26] *Walter vs. Baue* [27] involved a fourth-grade student injured while performing an experiment with rubber bands and a ruler detailed in his science textbook. He claimed the text was a defective product due to its failure to warn of the danger. Denying the plaintiff an action for products liability, the court plainly expressed its fears:

> The danger of plaintiff's proposed theory is the chilling effect it would have on the First Amendment Freedoms of Speech and Press. Would any author wish to be exposed to liability for writing on a topic which might result in physical injury? e.g., How to cut trees; How to keep bees?[28]

Quite incredibly, the court addresses a chilling effect on authors when it is protecting publishers. It does not address a public policy designed to encourage authorship while leaving authors vulnerable to suit.

Is Information Ever a Product?

Aetna Casualty & Surety Co. vs. Jeppesen & Co.[29] was a suit over an airline crash in Las Vegas against a publisher's graphic chart depiction of federal data for an instrument approach to the runway. The Ninth Circuit found the chart to be a "product." The chart translated data into a graphic portrayal. This holding dates to 1981, ten years before the same federal appellate court was so protective of mushroom guides in *Winter vs. G.P. Putnam's Sons.* In *Winter,* the Ninth Circuit distinguished mushroom guides from airplane charts saying:

> Aeronautical charts are highly technical tools. They are graphic depictions of technical, mechanical data. The best analogy to an aeronautical chart is a compass. Both may be used to guide an individual who is engaged in an activity requiring certain knowledge of natural features. Computer software that fails to yield the result for which it was designed may be another. In contrast, *The Encyclopedia of Mushrooms* is like a book on how to use a compass or an aeronautical chart. The chart itself is like a physical "product" while the "How to Use" book is pure thought and expression.[30]

This less than persuasive reasoning has been challenged by numerous authorities arguing that a mushroom book is as much a technical guide as an airplane chart; both are designed for those engaged in a hazardous activity. The danger of flawed information is real and substantial.[31] Having a cause of action for an exploding auto tire but not for false factual information in a mushroom book is more than an anomaly.

It simply defies logic. Moreover, the Appellate Court of Illinois, in considering whether an air conditioning system was a product once installed in a building, held that social policy justifications behind strict tort should be the guide rather than "a dictionary definition of the term 'product.'"[32] Public policy is one of loss allocation being placed on the sellers who are best able to organize their affairs and bear the cost.[33] This should serve as a low alarm for the scientific and medical publishing industry.

Alm vs. Van Nostrand Reinhold Co.[34] dealt with a victim of a shattered tool when he was following directions in *The Making of Tools*. With familiar reasoning, the court warned of a severe burden being laid on publishers of having to scrutinize and even test all procedures in their publications.[35] But the fact of the matter is that retailers do not test the products they sell in their stores. They buy products liability insurance. The objective of strict tort is to force the purchase of that insurance to put the spill-over cost of the injured consumer back on those making money from the product.

HAS ANYTHING CHANGED?

The law has not budged since these cases, which are all before the year 2000. What has changed radically is the nature of medical publishing. At first glance, this would appear to be untrue. Print is now delivered electronically. It is the same information. The law should be the same. But cybermedicine has spawned a multiplicity of technology-enabled interactions among health care providers and consumers/patients. Advice and content sites carry the risk of the Web site publishing its own advice or content and often guaranteeing this advice. These sites are unlike the traditional publisher whose materials are supplied by an author.

WebMD, for example, is a "provider of health information services to consumers, physicians, healthcare professionals, employers and health plans."[36] It claims not to provide medical advice or diagnosis, but the Web site has major health guides for symptoms, tests, and drugs. Advertising policy states that WebMD is not endorsing advertised products and is careful to distinguish advertisement from editorial. This would seem to protect them under the *Walters vs. Seventeen Magazine*[8] holding. But WebMD also states it will not accept ads that are not factually accurate. This statement sounds arguably like a guarantee. And all lawyers need is a basis for argument.

The Consumer and Patient Health Information Section (CAPHIS) of the Medical Library Association publishes a Top 100 "Web Sites You Can Trust." The stated purpose of the CAPHIS list is for the use of CAPHIS members and other librarians, yet anyone can access the site. At the bottom of the first screen, they disclaim any "direct recommendation or sponsorship" of any of the sites, emphasizing that some of the information is the "opinion of the author." And of course they throw in the standard "consult your healthcare provider."[37] Is this an adequate disclaimer, or could a lawyer pick at the bold-type endorsement at the top and the disclaimer way down at the bottom? It might be advisable to move the disclaimer up to the top and include some reference to the methodology of selecting the Top 100.

Blurring of Data and Product

Products liability for publishing has in large part been kept at bay by courts holding that information was not a product. Yet access to medical information is now widely obtained through multiple aggregators and search engines that are often marketed as electronic products. Some provide more than what is in a book or journal, adding, for example, links and video. Some advertise seamless integration between information and searching and browsing capabilities. Some are created and owned by publishers themselves. One could argue that tangible products are merging with ideas and information.

Many publishers or aggregators of electronic databases provide access to, or indexing of, medical information. In so doing, they are making decisions about what is important and how the content can or should be searched. In times past, a trained search analyst would craft the search with the help of a trained professional in the area. With search engines, metadata, and federated searching, much of this has been usurped by the machine or the humans who write the code behind the machine's retrieval base. One can argue, then, that data is becoming blurred by the product which is being offered on the market.

Aeronautical Charts Redux

Is MD Consult on all-fours with the aeronautical charts in *Aetna vs. Jeppeson?*[29] MD Consult is an Internet "service which combines an aggregation of clinical information resources, including … text books, fulltext journals, book series, clinical care guidelines, databases with links to fulltext, patient information, drug information, and current awareness resources."[38]

The Web site advertises that MD Consult provides "physicians step-by-step text and video demonstrations of commonly performed office procedures..." It promises improved physician productivity and improved patient care. It boasts "Short Answer, Long Answer ... Always the Right Answer."[39]

Remember that the airplane chart rationale was that the chart acts as the functional equivalent of products like a compass or navigational instrument. The chart information reaches beyond ideas to a representation of the data.[40] Is MD Consult a tool of such quality that doctors will be dubious about contradicting it? Does this have any impact on medical libraries? Going to the Web site of the Medical University of South Carolina,[41] one finds Consumer Health Topics with a subheading of, for example, Cancer. This gives you a link to Cancerquest,[42] which is supported by Emory University. The link states "[t]he target audience for our site includes cancer patients, their families and friends, medical workers and others interested in the subject,"[42] in other words, laypeople. The disclaimer reads like a contract with language such as, "you understand and agree that the information contained on this site is not intended nor implied to be, and you will not use it as a substitute for professional medical advice, diagnosis, or treatment."[42] While that is certainly a disclaimer and a strong warning to the consumer, it is not a contract. The reader does not have to click on an "I agree" to be able to access the information. The reader has demonstrated no acceptance of the terms of the offer nor even indicated having read them. And you have to click on "disclaimer" to read it. With a few clicks of the mouse, the reader has breezed through two medical university libraries and into information published by a medical group at Emory. This is a pretty good example of blurring data with product with publisher.

CONCLUSION

Lawyers are never reluctant to pursue to creative litigation and will certainly continue to bring suit against the publishing industry under new theories. No one has raised the question of whether rigorous refereeing is tantamount to an endorsement or guarantee. No one has tested the aeronautical chart holding on a case of erroneous data with built-in browsers. The good news for medical publishing is that it is not like manufacturing asbestos. The entire product is not poisonous; the entire industry cannot be taken down. Indeed, medical publishing has such high standards that at most only a tiny fraction of content might ever present a problem, but a problem that could nonetheless result in human illness or death. Given that potential damage, it seems likely that medical publishers will be buying products liability insurance in the near future. In the case of medical libraries, the crafting of highly visible and thorough disclaimers should prove adequate.

REFERENCES

1. Restatement (Second) of Torts § 283 (1965).
2. Heaven vs. Pender, 11 Q.B.D. 503, 509 (Q.B. 1883).
3. 833 P.2d 70 (Haw. 1992).
4. 833 P.2d at 75.
5. 694 F. Supp. 1216 (D. Md. 1988).
6. 694 F. Supp. at 1216, *See Lewin vs. McCreight,* 655 F. Supp. 282 (E.D. Mich. 1987); *Demuth Development Corp. vs. Merck & Co., Inc.,* 432 F. Supp. 990 (E.D.N.Y. 1977); *Alm vs. Van Nostrand Reinhold Co.,* 134 Ill. App. 3d 716, 480 N.E.2d 1263 (1985).
7. 694 F. Supp. at 1217.
8. 195 Cal. App. 3d 1119 (1987).
9. 195 Cal. App. 3d at 1121.
10. 195 Cal. App. at 1122.
11. (1969) 276 Cal.App.2d 680 [81 Cal.Rptr. 519, 39 A.L.R.3d 173].
12. 276 Cal. App.2d at 682.
13. 276 Cal. App.2d at 684.
14. *Walters vs. Seventeen*, 195 Cal.App.3d at 1122.
15. *See MacPherson vs. Buick Motor Co.,* 111 N.E. 1050 (N.Y. Ct. App. 1916) for the alleged origin of product liability law.
16. *Prosser & Keeton on the Law of Torts,* § 98, at 692-93 (W. Keeton ed. 5th ed. 1984); *Reilly vs. King County Central Blood Bank, Inc.,* 492 P.2d 246, 248 (Wash. 1971).
17. (1) One who sells any product in a defective condition unreasonably dangerous to the user or consumer or to his property is subject to liability for physical harm thereby caused to the ultimate user or consumer, or to his property, if (a) the seller is engaged in the business of selling such a product, and (b) it is expected to and does reach the user or consumer without substantial change in the condition in which it is sold. (2) The rule stated in Subsection (1) applies although (a) the seller has exercised all possible care in the preparation and sale of his product, and (b) the user or consumer has not bought the product from or entered into any contractual relation with the seller.
18. 27 Cal. Rptr. 697 (Cal. 1963).
19. *American Law of Products Liability* 3D §§ 1:25-29 (1987).
20. 386 Pa. Super. 392, 563 A.2d 123 (Pa. Super. Ct. 1989).
21. 386 Pa. Super. at 398. *See Herceg vs. Hustler Magazine, Inc.,* 565 F.Supp. 802 (S.D. Texas 1983).

22. 342 So.2d 1053 (Fla.Dist.Ct.App.1977).

23. 342 So.2d at 1056.

24. 938 F.2d 1033 (9th Cir. 1991).

25. 938 F.2d at 1035.

26. 694 F. Supp. at 1217. *See Gertz vs. Robert Welch, Inc.*, 418 U.S. 323, 41 L. Ed. 2d 789, 94 S. Ct. 2997 (1974).

27. 439 N.Y.S.2d 821 (N.Y. Sup. Ct. 1981), *aff'd in part & rev'd in part on other grounds*, 88 A.D.2d 787 (N.Y. App Div. 1982).

28. 439 N.Y.S.2d at 822-23.

29. 642 F.2d 339 (9th Cir. 1981).

30. 938 F.2d at 1035.

31. Arnold, Roy W. "The Persistence of Caveat Emptor: Publisher Immunity from Liability for Inaccurate Factual Information." *University of Pittsburgh Law Review* 53(Spring 1992): 777.

32. *London Trent vs. Brasch Manufacturing Company, Inc., et al.*, 132 Ill. App. 3d 586, 589; 477 N.E.2d 1312, 1315 (1985).

33. *Restatement (Second) of Torts* § 402A; Mintz, Jonathan B. "Strict Liability for Commercial Intellect." *Catholic University Law Review* 41(1992): 617,632.

34. 480 N.E.2d 1263 (Ill. App. Ct. 1985).

35. 480 N.E.2d at 1267.

36. WebMD. Available: <http://www.webmd.com>. Accessed: September 8, 2006.

37. Consumer and Patient Health Information Section. Available: <http://caphis. mlanet.org/consumer/index.html>. Accessed: September 15, 2006.

38. MDConsult Review. *The Charleston Advisor* 1(July 1999): 16.

39. MDConsult. Available: <http://www.mdconsult.com/>. Accessed: September 8, 2006.

40. 938 F.2d at 1036; 694 F. Supp. at 1217.

41. Medical University of South Carolina. Available: <http://www.library.musc.edu/>. Accessed: September 8, 2006.

42. Cancerquest. Available: <http://www.cancerquest.org/>. Accessed: September 8, 2006.

doi:10.1300/J383v04n01_10

Semantic Web Technologies:
Opportunity for Domain Targeted Libraries?

Jon C. Ferguson

SUMMARY. The World Wide Web has become a compelling mechanism for access to medical libraries and evidence-based databases. However, the current Web lacks the Semantic machinery to expose and reason with detailed knowledge. The Semantic Web can provide this by making formal knowledge available across Web sites, creating opportunities for collaborative discovery. This article discusses emerging Semantic Web technologies and how they can be applied to digital libraries. Examples are drawn from cross-disciplinary research into maternal health in developing nations being conducted by IMMPACT (The Initiative for Maternal Mortality Programme Assessment). doi:10.1300/J383v04n01_11 *[Article copies available for a fee from The Haworth Document Delivery Service: 1-800-HAWORTH. E-mail address: <docdelivery@haworthpress.com> Website: <http://www.HaworthPress.com> © 2007 by The Haworth Press, Inc. All rights reserved.]*

Jon C. Ferguson, PhD, was Senior Health Database Scientist for the IMMPACT project, Department of Health, University of Aberdeen, Foresterhill Lea, Westburn Road, Aberdeen, United Kingdom AB25 2ZL. Dr. Ferguson is currently affiliated with Digital Steps Limited (jon.ferguson@digitalsteps.com).

This work was undertaken as part of an international research programme–IMMPACT (Initiative for Maternal Mortality Programme Assessment <http://www.abdn.ac.uk/immpact>), funded by the Bill & Melinda Gates Foundation, Department for International Development, European Commission, and USAID. The funders have no responsibility for the information provided or views expressed in this article. The views expressed herein are solely those of the author.

[Haworth co-indexing entry note]: "Semantic Web Technologies: Opportunity for Domain Targeted Libraries?" Ferguson, Jon C. Co-published simultaneously in the *Journal of Electronic Resources in Medical Libraries* (The Haworth Information Press, an imprint of The Haworth Press, Inc.) Vol. 4, No. 1/2, 2007, pp. 113-125; and: *Electronic Resources in Medical Libraries: Issues and Solutions* (ed: Elizabeth Connor, and M. Sandra Wood) The Haworth Information Press, an imprint of The Haworth Press, Inc., 2007, pp. 113-125. Single or multiple copies of this article are available for a fee from The Haworth Document Delivery Service [1-800-HAWORTH, 9:00 a.m. - 5:00 p.m. (EST). E-mail address: docdelivery@haworthpress.com].

KEYWORDS. Ontology, taxonomy, Semantic Web, knowledge management, domain specific libraries, maternal health

INTRODUCTION

The current Web is truly a "disruptive technology," as it has drastically lowered the cost of entry to publishing information to a potentially huge audience. The ability to dynamically generate Web pages from database silos has led to the proliferation of online databases and the ability to search library resources from across the globe. Libraries are going digital, and as a result, researchers spend less time onsite within library buildings.

Regardless, the conventional Web has acted mostly like a window onto conventional library databases. The Web interface was just that: a presentation of abstracts and papers with facilities to enter searches to the underlying database engine. Sitting in a server room somewhere was software which would perform the query on the database and present the results using the hypertext markup language (HTML). HTML, derived from the more powerful standard generalized markup language (SGML), has always been a presentation language–its strength has been its simplicity and ability to link pages together. Unfortunately what it does not do well is separate knowledge from presentation. As librarians know, indexing is about knowledge. Keywords are used to capture key concepts discussed in a paper, even if the exact keyword is not present in the text itself. Concepts may be represented by several words. Concepts also depend on context: a "jaguar" may be an animal or a car.

This is nothing new to librarians since classifications, controlled vocabularies, and thesauri (Dewey Decimal System, Medical Subject Headings, Unified Medical Language System) have been used for years to index library content. Medical libraries have been especially adept at classifying complex information. What is new is that these concepts have been externalized and enriched by the Web medium to make search and machine inference possible. In effect, Web 1.0 lacks the Semantic machinery to clearly externalize the knowledge and relationships captured in myriad databases. To quote a well-worn statement, "If HTML and the Web made all the online documents look like one huge book, RDF, schema, and inference languages will make all the data in the world look like one huge database."[1] This is the goal of the Semantic Web.

The Semantic Web approach has the potential to be powerful for three reasons. First, it helps to formalize concepts and relationships to enhance machine understanding which in turn can be used to perform several tasks, such as reasoning over medical evidence[2,3,4] or enhancing searching.[5] Second, it fosters a shared understanding of the knowledge domains across diverse groups of people; a conceptual model can be viewed and analyzed, revealing underlying assumptions and relationships between important concepts. Third, it provides an opportunity for knowledge linking and collaboration across databases and knowledge domains and increases opportunities for discovery.[6,7] It should be clear that the Semantic Web will not replace medical databases but rather augment, unite, and make them more accessible.

Others have provided an overview of Semantic Web technologies and their use in several applications handling medical information.[8] The goal of this article is to investigate opportunities for domain-targeted digital libraries and discuss the potential for connecting resources across repositories and collaborating knowledge domains. Examples are drawn from cross-disciplinary research into maternal health in developing nations being conducted by IMMPACT (The Initiative for Maternal Mortality Programme Assessment), which combines several knowledge domains: obstetrics, economics, policy, and health systems, to name a few.

To begin with, there is a need to highlight the utility of ontology languages, specifically the Web Ontology Language (OWL), for building rich conceptual models that can be shared across the Web. Subject terms, such as medical subject headings (MeSH), can be used to link research papers to taxonomies in research libraries. A subject term is effectively part of a controlled vocabulary that is understood in light of the standardized "offline" MeSH conceptual model. OWL can provide for a richer conceptual model but also leverages ideas from Web 1.0 that effectively allow unequivocal connection to be made between the "offline" conceptual model and the "keyword" annotation of the paper.

WHAT MAKES ONTOLOGIES DIFFERENT?

There have been many definitions of ontologies,[9] but most involve a formal, shared conceptual model of a knowledge domain of interest. In practical terms, "An ontology typically consists of a hierarchical description of important concepts in a domain, along with descriptions of the properties of each concept, and constraints about these concepts and properties."[10] Thus, an ontology is more expansive than a taxonomy, which is usually a hierarchical model, in that it can include properties or attributes of the concepts included in the hierarchy as well as specified constraints. Properties are descriptive: *has-color, is-related-to, has-author, causes*, etc. They can be used to relate individuals to individuals (where an *individual* is an example of a concept) or values to concept/individuals such as "Joe is-related-to Pam," or "Kettle has-color black." In these cases, Joe and Pam are examples of the concept *Person* and *Kettle* is a concept in a kitchen ontology. Note that the lines between Individuals and Concepts are a bit blurred and model dependent. A *Kettle* could also be an individual example of a *CookingUtensil* concept. *ElectricKettle* could be an individual example of the *Kettle* concept, as could *KettleNo3*. Concepts are collections of Individuals; that is, they classify them.

In another example, the knowledge domain might be *safe motherhood* and could include concepts such as *Maternal Mortality, Maternal Mortality Ratio* (MMR), *Lifetime risk of maternal death*, and the five major direct causes of maternal death in developing countries. Figure 1 shows a partial ontology based on some of these concepts and modeled using the Protégé modeling tool.[11]

On the face of it, this ontology could be considered a taxonomy, meaning a simple classification of concepts. However as mentioned above, an ontology can have properties. For example, both pre-eclampsia and eclampsia are types of hypertension. However, pre-eclampsia may or may not lead to eclampsia, and eclampsia is effectively characterized by convulsions. This can be modeled by adding a property *has-precursor* linking eclampsia to preeclampsia (not shown in Figure 1). Another property *has-clinical-sign* is used to link clinical signs (for which a partial hierarchy is shown) to medical conditions (e.g., *pre-eclampsia has-clinical-sign Proteinuria*). In ontologies, links are not just hierarchical (*is_a*) or containership (*has_a*) relationships.

Furthermore, concepts in ontologies can carry assertions. Assertions formally define restrictions on relationships (e.g., a *Mother* must have had at least one *Child* and must be a *Female*). In this example, these are used to add characteristics to concepts that can be used for automated classification. Running the reasoner from within Protégé results in the following *inferred* concept hierarchy (see Figure 2). As mentioned, both *Pre-Eclampsia* and *Eclampsia* are types of Hypertension, but simultaneously each is also a *MaternalComplication*. The reasoner (RacerPro <http://www.racer-systems.com>) determines from the properties attached to *Eclampsia* and *Pre-Eclampsia* that they are also subsumed by sub-types of *Hypertension*. A similar automatic classification

FIGURE 1. A Simple Ontology (Asserted)

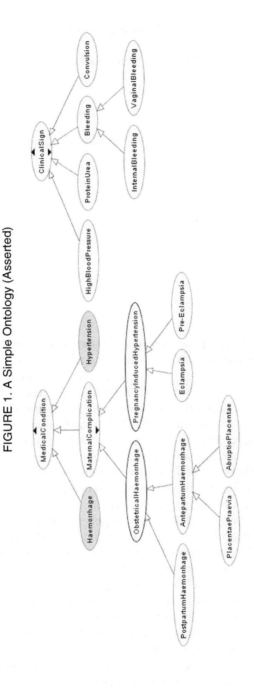

FIGURE 2. A Simple Ontology (Inferred)

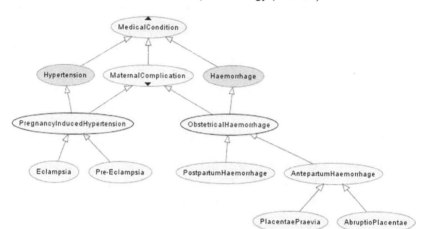

happens with *Haemorrhage* and *ObstetricalHaemorrhage*. Semantic searching is enhanced by these asserted and inferred relationships since a search for *Haemorrhage* in the context of maternal death should return results related to *ObstetricHaemorrhage*. Furthermore, the ontology can model the causal link between another concept: *UterineRupture* and *Haemorrhage*. Such causal knowledge can be used to enable researchers to search for examples of conditions (uterine rupture, etc.) that might contribute to a regional incidence of hemorrhage.

Rich conceptual models allow more to be said about the content of a document and how this content may fit into the target domain of interest. In building a knowledge base of evidence or mapping a library of documents containing evidence, it is important to build conceptual models that are appropriate to the task. For example, in IMMPACT, the task has been to build a sustainable evidence base that links papers and evidence for public health researchers and policy makers to understand the drivers for safe motherhood in developing countries. The conceptual models must therefore include some aspects on the medical causes of maternal death, as shown above, but they must also include other aspects such as transport issues (a hemorrhaging mother needs treatment within a particular time period and must be able to get to the hospital), and of health systems (mapping capabilities and services offered at different hospitals and health facilities), among other things.

As a result, there is a need to work with several conceptual models together. Thankfully, Web ontology languages have been built with this requirement in mind and therefore provide the tools to accomplish this task. The value of combining several conceptual models together is shown in the example of modeling Comprehensive Emergency Care Facilities using a definition put forward by the United Nations Population Fund (UNFPA)[12] and linking them to *Individual* facilities that are mapped using global positioning systems (see Figure 3).

FIGURE 3. Simple Health Service Model with Global Positioning Systems

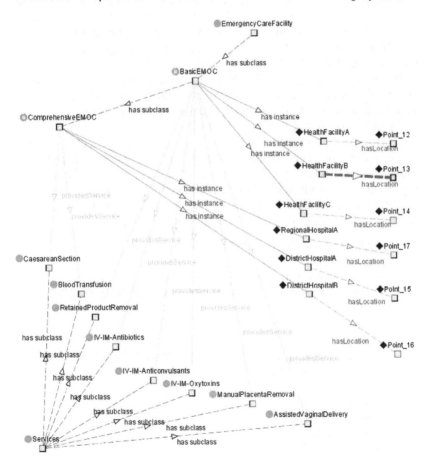

In the first conceptual model, a basic Emergency Obstetric Care (EmOC) facility must be able to provide six important services, whereas a comprehensive EmOC facility needs to perform surgery (Caesarean section) and blood transfusion in addition to these basic services (services are located in the bottom left corner of Figure 3). The second conceptual model (right side of the figure) introduces geographical coordinates by making use of the "geo" ontology based on the resource description framework (RDF) from the World Wide Web Consortium (<http://www.w3.org/2003/01/geo>, where the RDF file is at <http://www.w3.org/2003/01/geo/wgs84_pos#>). This simple vocabulary defines a *SpatialThing* base concept from which *Point* is derived. It also defines *lat, long, lat_long,* and *alt* properties. For simplicity, only individual *Point*s are shown in the figure but their details are highlighted in the extensible markup language (XML) text in the next paragraph, which states that "Health Facility A" is a basic emergency care facility located at latitude 12.333 degrees and longitude 0.955 degrees.

In the model, a regional hospital is assumed to provide comprehensive EmOC services as does a district hospital. Some health centers provide basic EmOC. As it turns out, there are country-specific aspects of the health system that will vary, and whether a hospital really provides the full set of comprehensive EmOC services is dependent on staffing levels at the time. This highlights the use of *Individuals* to map the hospitals and health centers. Concepts (or Classes) such as *BasicEmOC* represent sets of Individuals. Individuals in this case therefore represent specific facilities (*HealthFacilityA*) that can be found on the map, hence the geo:lat/geo:long use from the imported ontology:

```
<BasicEMOC rdf:ID="HealthFacilityA">
  <hasLocation>
    <geo:Point rdf:ID="Point_1">
      <geo:lat rdf:datatype="http://www.w3.org/2001/XMLSchema#
      string">
        12.333
      </geo:lat>
      <geo:long rdf:datatype="http://www.w3.org/2001/XML
      Schema#string">
        0.955
      </geo:long>
    </geo:Point>
  </hasLocation>
</BasicEMOC>
```

OWL does not use the so-called Unique Name Assumption (UNA), so it is quite possible to manage multiple documents referring to the same facility by different names.[13] Reasoning allows the program to imply that the names all refer to the same facility. For example, it could be said that the property *hasLocation* is Functional, that is, any Basic-EMOC at a particular point (defined by lat/long/alt) is the same, regardless of the name given to the facility. Since this knowledge may have been extracted from different documents or other knowledge sources, it provides a logical way to build up information about a particular facility from disparate fragments.

The Semantic Web can work with knowledge from different sources to form a kind of distributed and sustainable knowledge base. The implications could be quite powerful for domain-specific libraries—or even libraries that support annotation using shared ontologies. These implications have been highlighted about the Semantic Web in general.[14] A dynamic demonstration of using geographic location to link disparate information can be seen at <http://geoURL.org>. This site merely indexes Web pages according to location information and provides a map interface to find the links. It would be much more valuable for a search to semantically link libraries from well-known sources using ontologies that were complementary to a domain of interest.

A final important aspect that makes ontologies so powerful is that by modeling concepts rather than just classifying them, there is the possibility to minimize the combinatorial explosion that results in large attempts at classification, especially in regard to medical terminologies.[15] Generalized Architecture for Languages, Encyclopedias, and Nomenclatures in Medicine (GALEN) is an example of such an approach.

LINKING THE CONCEPTUAL MODEL TO CONTENT

The Semantic Web encourages traceability between conceptual models and the use of their concepts in publications. The genius of Tim Berners-Lee's vision of the Web is that HTML has the syntactic machinery in the form of uniform resource identifiers (URIs) and uniform resource locators (URLs) to link almost anything, making traceability possible. References to the ontology model in use as well as respective annotations can be made either inside the Web page itself (within metatags for example) or via an included RDF file.

Alternatively, knowledge can be "overlaid" on an original Web page by use of an "annotation server" such as Annotea <http://www.w3.org/

2001/Annotea/>. Kampa et al.[7] made use of this approach to enable the application of knowledge-based markup to views of presented documents. They modeled the relationships between the literature, authors, and project teams and used this knowledge to superimpose links to discovered relationships such as other papers written by the author, researchers working on the same project, etc., onto the original document. In this approach, the conceptual model is completely separate from the original document–URIs/URLs are used to dynamically link the model, original document, and any discovered annotations.

CHALLENGES:
CAPTURING CONCEPTS–SHARING KNOWLEDGE

The strength of a particular ontology is related to its detail and the size of its user base. Obtaining agreement within a user group on which particular concepts to use and what exactly they mean is not easy. The larger the user base, the harder this is. Furthermore, it appears that the larger the user base, the less detailed the ontology is likely to be. It is easier to obtain agreement on general concepts. As a result, there are efforts to enable translation between ontologies. One such approach is called "Semantic Negotiation."[16] Others have investigated linking common concepts among ontologies.[17] Borrowing from database modeling concepts, this could almost be called a "Semantic foreign keys" approach to linking ontologies by providing a way to reject concepts from inappropriate ontologies. For example, when looking for big Jaguar cats, a car ontology is rejected even though Jaguar is a concept used.

Some domains (such as safe motherhood) represent a relatively small set of experts. In smaller domains, it should be possible to agree on a more detailed ontology that would be capable of more detailed statements, although linking information among various specific areas (medical, transport, health services, as mentioned before) is part of the challenge.

Another issue is how to index a large set of relevant documents using such a detailed ontology. Quality detailed indexing is costly and generally requires highly skilled personnel.[18] Furthermore, any evolutionary changes in the ontology can be problematic since re-indexing would be necessary. On the other hand, several researchers are attempting large-scale automated indexing.[19-21] These efforts generally utilize some form of natural language processing (NLP). Despite great improvements, NLP generally cannot tag documents with deep ontological concepts.

Furthermore, they do need large control sets of consistent documents for training the algorithms.

Perhaps the community of users can address this challenge by using a combination of automated and manual methods. An interface could be used to allow community members to annotate deep concepts in resources based on a common requirement to understand a particular domain, thereby leading to knowledge discovery through analysis. The approach could be further augmented if stakeholders require publications to be annotated at the time of submission.

CONCLUSION

What will be the impact of the Semantic Web on library technology? Others have already reported a large increase in online usage of library material.[22] Use of ontologies within medicine is well established. The Web's strengths include its simplicity, ease of use, and ubiquity for collaboration even though it also can be seen to trivialize information and opens up issues of trust and reliability. The Semantic Web carries the potential to bring clarity and reliability to Web content. Development of shared ontologies is challenging but smaller communities such as the "Safe Motherhood" research community can be targeted. In this way, ontologies can be augmentative–providing deeper modeling and reasoning possibilities for more specific domains. Funders in these particular domains can help the drive toward proper annotation at the point of publication and these annotations can be incorporated into online documents. The result would be distribution of costs related to annotation while improving understanding of the domain by new researchers, allowing Semantic searching, and providing better opportunities for automated reasoning and domain modeling. Domains such as "Safe Motherhood" could lead to evidence-adaptive policy decision support systems. Sim et al.[3] discuss adaptive clinical decision support systems.

Significant enhancements will be necessary to achieve these goals. Specifically, the following issues need to be addressed:

- Current reasoning is slow over large knowledge bases, although these capabilities can be significantly enhanced by making use of offline reasoning and indexing services.
- Ontology creation is difficult due to the need for wide collaboration in order to build an acceptable and clear, formal definition that is suitable for various purposes. Large ontologies struggle to keep the combinatorial explosion under control. This can be addressed

by developing better methods to partition large ontologies and re-use a combination of smaller ones.

* Annotation costs are high if accomplished by hand; current automated methods cannot cope with deeply nested ontologies or concept properties. Some progress is being made with NLP-based approaches[20] and the extraction of relationships through the use of carefully constructed user interfaces.[23] Taking advantage of collaboration in online communities is another way to capture rich annotation while promoting knowledge discovery, if community engagement can be achieved.

REFERENCES

1. Berners-Lee, Tim, and Fischetti, Mark. *Weaving the Web: The Original Design and Ultimate Destiny of the World Wide Web.* New York: HarperCollins, 1999.

2. Sim, Ida. *Trial Banks: An Informatics Foundation for Evidence-Based Medicine.* Ph.D. dissertation, Stanford University, 1997.

3. Sim, Ida; Gorman, Paul; Greenes, Robert A. et al. "Clinical Decision Support Systems for the Practice of Evidence-based Medicine." *Journal of the American Medical Informatics Association* 8, no. 6 (2001): 527-34.

4. Sim, Ida; Sanders, Gillian D.; and McDonald, Kathryn M. "Evidence-based Practice for Mere Mortals: The Role of Informatics and Health Services Research." *Journal of General Internal Medicine* 17, no. 4 (2002): 302-8.

5. McGuinness, Deborah L. "Ontology-Enhanced Search for Primary Care Medical Literature." In: *Proceedings of the International Medical Informatics Association Working Group 6 on Medical Concept Representation and Natural Language Processing Conference*, Phoenix, Arizona, December 16-19, 1999.

6. Carr, L.; Kampa, S.; De Roure, D. et al. "Ontological Linking: Motivation and Analysis." Available: <http://cohse.semanticweb.org/papers/cikm.doc>. Accessed: July 28, 2006.

7. Kampa, S.; Miles-Board, T.; Carr, L.; and Hall, W. "Linking with Meaning: Ontological Hypertext for Scholars." Technical Report ECSTR-IAM01-005, Electronics and Computer Science, University of Southampton, 2001. Available: <http://www.kampa.org/papers/lwm.pdf>. Accessed: July 28, 2006.

8. Robu, I.; Robu, V.; and Thirion, B. "An Introduction to the Semantic Web for Health Sciences Librarians." *Journal of the Medical Library Association* 94, no. 2 (2006):198-205.

9. Fensel, Dieter; Hendler, James A.; Lieberman, Henry; and Wahlster, Wolfgang. "Introduction." In: *Spinning the Semantic Web*, edited by Dieter Fensel, James Hendler, Henry Lieberman, and Wolfgang Wahlster, 1-25. Cambridge, MA: The MIT Press, 2003.

10. Pan, Jeff Z. *Description Logics: Reasoning Support for the Semantic Web.* Ph.D. dissertation, University of Manchester, 2004.

11. The Protégé Ontology Editor and Knowledge Acquisitions System [database online]. Stanford Medical Informatics, Stanford University School of Medicine. Available: <http://protege.stanford.edu>. Accessed: July 28, 2006.

12. Emergency Obstetric Care Checklist for Planners. United Nations Population Fund (UNFPA) [database online]. Available: <http://www.unfpa.org/upload/lib_pub_file/150_filename_checklist_MMU.pdf>. Accessed: July 28, 2006.

13. Horridge, Matthew; Knublauch, Holger; Rector, Alan; Stevens, Robert; and Wroe, Chris. *A Practical Guide to Building OWL Ontologies Using the Protégé-OWL Plugin and CO-ODE Tools, Edition 1.0.* Available: <http://www.co-ode.org/resources/tutorials/ProtegeOWLTutorial.pdf>. Accessed: July 28, 2006.

14. Hendler, Jim. "From Atoms to OWLs: The New Ecology of the WWW." Keynote speech presented at XML 2005 Conference & Exposition, Atlanta, GA, November 14-18, 2005. Available: <http://www.cs.umd.edu/~hendler/presentations/XML2005Keynote.pdf>. Accessed: July 28, 2006.

15. Rector, Alan. "Semantic Webs and the Semantic Web: Services, Resources and Technologies for Clinical Care and Biomedical Research." Paper presented at the 15th International World Wide Web Conference, Edinburgh, Scotland, May 23-26, 2006. Available: <http://www2006.org/speakers/rector/rector.ppt>. Accessed: July 28, 2006.

16. Guha, R., and McCool, R. "TAP: A Semantic Web Platform." *Computer Networks* 42, no. 5 (2003): 557-77.

17. Arumugam, M.; Sheth, A.; and Arpinar, I. "Towards Peer-to-Peer Semantic Web: A Distributed Environment for Sharing Semantic Knowledge on the Web." In: *Proceedings of WWW-02 Workshop on Real World RDF and Semantic Web Applications*, Honolulu, HI, May 7, 2002.

18. Ward, Rod. "Human Quality Assurance for Web Resource Catalogues." Paper presented at the 15th International World Wide Web Conference, Edinburgh, Scotland, May 23-26, 2006. Available: <http://www2006.org/speakers/ward/ward.pdf>. Accessed: July 28, 2006.

19. Ciravegna, Fabio; Chapman, Sam; Dingli, Alexiei; and Wilks, Yorick. "Learning to Harvest Information for the Semantic Web." In: *Proceedings of the 1st European Semantic Web Symposium*, Heraklion, Greece, May 10-12, 2004. Available: <http://eprints.pascal-network.org/archive/00000918/>. Accessed: July 28, 2006.

20. Dill, S.; Eiron, N.; Gibson, D. et al. *SemTag and Seeker: Bootstrapping the Semantic Web via Automated Semantic Annotation.* Paper presented at the 12th International World Wide Web Conference, Budapest, Hungary, May 20-24, 2003. Available: <http://www2003.org/cdrom/papers/refereed/p831/p831-dill.html>. Accessed: July 28, 2006.

21. Sheth, Amit, and Ramakrishnan, Cartic. "Semantic (Web) Technology in Action: Ontology Driven Information Systems for Search, Integration and Analysis." *IEEE Data Engineering Bulletin* 26, no. 4 (2003): 40-8.

22. Gentry, Mark, and Marone, R. Kenny. "The Virtual Medical Library: Resources at the Point of Need via a Proxy Server." *Journal of Electronic Resources in Medical Libraries* 1, no. 1 (2004): 3-20.

23. Bosman, B., and Droogmans, L. "Conversion and Metadata Extraction Frameworks." Paper presented at DSpace Federation 2nd User Group Meeting, Cambridge, England, July 6-8, 2005.

doi:10.1300/J383v04n01_11

Index